Mycotoxins and Food Safety - Recent Advances

Edited by Romina Alina Marc

Published in London, United Kingdom

Mycotoxins and Food Safety - Recent Advances
http://dx.doi.org/10.5772/intechopen.95720
Edited by Romina Alina Marc

Contributors
Lídia Palma, Paula Pereira, Marisa Nicolai, Azhar A. Alhaddad, Romina Alina Marc, Elie Fereche Itoba-Tombo, Seteno Karabo Obed Ntwampe, John Baptist Nzukizi Mudumbi, Lukhanyo Mekuto, Enoch Akinbiyi Akinbiyi Akinpelu, Nkosikho Dlangamandla, Hsiu-Ling Chen, Rachelle D. Arcega, Samuel Herianto, Chih-Yao Hou, Chia-Min Lin, Zacharia Waithaka Ng'ang'a, Eric Niyonshuti, Dewi Susanna, Tris Eryando, Budi Hartono, Lassie Fitria

First published in London, United Kingdom, 2022 by IntechOpen
IntechOpen is the global imprint of INTECHOPEN LIMITED, registered in England and Wales, registration number: 11086078, 5 Princes Gate Court, London, SW7 2QJ, United Kingdom

British Library Cataloguing-in-Publication Data
A catalogue record for this book is available from the British Library

Additional hard and PDF copies can be obtained from orders@intechopen.com

Mycotoxins and Food Safety - Recent Advances
Edited by Romina Alina Marc
p. cm.
Print ISBN 978-1-83962-903-7
Online ISBN 978-1-83962-904-4
eBook (PDF) ISBN 978-1-83962-918-1

Meet the editor

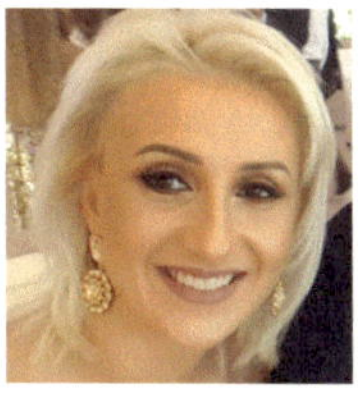

Romina Alina Marc (née Vlaic) obtained her Ph.D. in Agronomy at the University of Agricultural Sciences and Veterinary Medicine (UASVM) of Cluj-Napoca, Romania, in 2015. She is a lecturer and researcher in vegetable food quality control, rheology in the food industry, quality management systems, and food safety in the Faculty of Food Science and Technology, UASVM Cluj-Napoca. She has edited one book and published more than fifty manuscripts, four book chapters, and two books. She has participated in more than fifty international conferences and has won twenty-eight international awards and fourteen projects (seven as project director).

Contents

Preface

Today, consumers demand safe, minimally processed foods without microbiological hazards and additives but with a long shelf life. Food security is the basis of human health and quality of life. Today, global food security has become a major strategic issue and has attracted worldwide attention.

Food safety is achieved when food is available and accessible and when food use and stability are at levels that allow all people physical and economical access to affordable, safe, and nutritious food. When one of these four pillars weakens, then a society undermines its food security.

Most countries have established laws and regulations to provide the population with safe food. According to the law, safe food is non-toxic, harmless, and in accordance with nutritional requirements. It does not pose acute, chronic, or potential danger to human health, for example, during planting, breeding, processing, packaging, storage, transport, sales, consumption, and other food activities. According to mandatory standards and requirements, there should be no foods that contain harmful or poisonous substances with hidden potential to cause harm or even death to consumers.

Food safety and quality are greatly influenced by pollution and economic development. Given the rapid socioeconomic changes of the last decade, food processing, food supply, and consumption patterns have undergone significant changes, increasing the number of food security problems. One of these problems, present worldwide, is mycotoxin contamination. This contamination decreases product quality and reduces export values, which can lead to significant economic losses for producing countries.

Mycotoxin contamination can be mitigated to acceptable levels through an integrated management approach along value chains, good agricultural practices, biological control, sorting, electromagnetic radiation treatments, ozone fumigation, chemical control agents, plant growth, good manufacturing practices, and Hazard Analysis Critical Control Point (HACCP) and other management systems used to reduce and prevent the risks of mycotoxin contamination. Contamination of food by mycotoxins has a considerable impact on food security, trade, economy, and public health.

Given the ongoing evolution in the field of food safety, this book, *Mycotoxins and Food Safety - Recent Advances*, presents comprehensive information on and recent advances in mycotoxins and food safety. aims to come up with the most comprehensive presentation of current information in the literature to improve existing knowledge about regards Recent Advances in Mycotoxins and Food Safety. Chapters are organized into the following five sections: "Introduction: Mycotoxins and Food Safety Overview"; "The Influence of Contaminants on Food Safety" "Mycotoxins in Feed"; "Indirect Mycotoxin Contamination of Food Safety"; and "Control and Reduction of Mycotoxin Contamination."

I would like to thank Author Service Managers Ms. Iva Simcic, Ms. Marijana Josipovic, and Ms. Ana Javor, at IntechOpen for their support during the preparation and publication of this book. I would also like to thank the contributing authors for their excellent chapters. I am especially grateful to my husband and children for their understanding and my colleagues at the University of Agricultural Sciences and Veterinary Medicine Cluj-Napoca for their support.

Romina Alina Marc
Food Engineering Department,
Faculty of Food Science and Technology,
University of Agricultural Sciences and Veterinary Medicine Cluj-Napoca,
Cluj Napoca, Romania

Section 1

Introduction: Mycotoxins and Food Safety Overview

Chapter 1

Implications of Mycotoxins in Food Safety

Romina Alina Marc

Abstract

The chapter aims to address an overview of the implications of mycotoxins in food safety and the presence of mycotoxins in various foods. Nowadays, everyone wants safe food with a long shelf life. Food safety has become a major strategic issue worldwide and has attracted worldwide attention. Mycotoxins are widely found in food and feed, and dietary exposure to them can induce various types of adverse health effects in humans and animals. Contamination of food by fungi and mycotoxins results in loss of dry matter, quality and nutrition, and poses a significant danger to the food chain. Moreover, mycotoxin contamination decreases product quality and reduces export values, which can lead to significant economic losses for producing countries. Mycotoxin contamination directly reduces food availability and has its own contribution to hunger and malnutrition, and the consumption of food contaminated with mycotoxins has major repercussions on human health.

Keywords: mycotoxins, food safety, aflatoxin, ochratoxins, zearalenone, fumonisin, patulin

1. Introduction

Food security is the basis of human health and quality of life. Today, food safety has become a major strategic issue in the world and has attracted worldwide attention [1].

Food security is effectively realized when food pillars, including food availability, access to food, food use, and food stability are at levels that allow all people to have physical and economical access to affordable, safe, and nutritious food to meet the requirement for a living active and healthy. When one of these four pillars weakens, then a society undermines its food security [2].

Most countries have established laws and regulations to provide the population with safe food. A safe food according to the law is nontoxic, harmless, and in accordance with nutritional requirements. It will not cause an acute, chronic, and potential danger to human health, for example, during planting, breeding, processing, packaging, storage, transport, sales, consumption, and other food activities. According to mandatory standards and requirements, there should be no foods with potential harm or danger to human health, such as harmful or poisonous substances with hidden potential to cause harm to consumers, which can lead to death [3].

Even though we have so much information at our disposal, the situation regarding global food security is still grim. Worldwide, food security and safety issues have increased over the past two decades. These increases continually raise questions about whether these current regulatory and control systems are effective. Recently, the World Health Organization (WHO), the Codex Alimentarius Commission (CAC), and other organizations have developed new limits for the safety of the international food trade [3].

Food safety and quality are greatly influenced by the living conditions of pollution in different countries, as well as their economic development. Given the rapid socio-economic changes of the last decade, worldwide, which promise a flourishing economic rise, food processing, food supply, and consumption patterns have undergone significant changes, increasing the number of outbreaks of food security problems. One of these problems, present worldwide, is given by mycotoxins [3].

Mycotoxins are one of the most important contributing factors to food loss, especially in developing countries, and have become a recurring challenge for food safety [4]. As a result, to date, serious concerns are raised by both consumers and health and nutrition professionals about the presence of mycotoxins in food [5]. Contamination of food by fungi and mycotoxins results in loss of dry matter, quality and nutrition, and poses a significant danger to the food chain [6].

Moreover, mycotoxin contamination decreases product quality and reduces export values, which can lead to significant economic losses for producing countries. Mycotoxin contamination directly reduces food availability and has its own contribution to hunger and malnutrition [4]. Drought stress, failure to implement good agricultural practices, poor postharvest practices, and insect infestation are factors that influence mycotoxin contamination [7, 8].

In addition, socio-economic factors, such as poor transport and trading systems, lack of awareness, and insufficient regulations and legislation, can also contribute to the risks of mycotoxin contamination [4].

Mycotoxin contamination can be mitigated to acceptable levels through an integrated management approach along value chains [2] good agricultural practices, biological control, sorting, electromagnetic radiation treatments, ozone fumigation, chemical control agents [2] plant growth [9], good manufacturing practices, Hazard Analysis Critical Control Point (HACCP), and others [4] are some of the methods used to reduce/prevent the risks of mycotoxin contamination.

Contamination of food and food by mycotoxins has a considerable impact on food insecurity, trade, economy, and public health [10].

Food safety and security are basic needs for consumers. The major goal of world organizations is to take action to ensure food safety and security. In addition to food, the consumer is also exposed to water through oral intake, to the environment through inhalation, and exposure of the skin and penetration through it. Consumption of foods contaminated with mycotoxins, mainly cereals and foods of animal origin, is the most important and common route of exposure. Mycotoxins found in animal feed can indeed be transported in animal tissues, especially the liver, kidneys, and eggs [11].

2. Generalities. short classification of the main mycotoxins involved in food safety

Mycotoxins contribute significantly to food loss in developing countries [2]. According to the Food and Agriculture Organization (FAO), about a third of total food is lost, totaling about 1.3 billion tons per year. It is also estimated that approximately five billion people worldwide are exposed to mycotoxins, such as aflatoxins. However, formulas for assessing the global economic impact of the presence of mycotoxins in food have been extremely difficult to develop [12]. Mycotoxins are a global public health problem, with spices, crops, meat, and dairy products being the main sources of mycotoxins [13].

The economic and social impact of these mycotoxins includes losses caused by death and disease of humans and animals, veterinary and medical costs, reduced animal productivity, loss of livelihoods, control measures, economic losses for farmers through food and feed losses, and waste due to contamination. The negative effects of mycotoxin exposure could be mitigated through the use of agricultural knowledge and public health practices, such as proper processing and storage of products [2, 12].

The problem of mycotoxins is of paramount importance because it can have carcinogenic, immunological, allergenic effects [14], toxigenic, nephrotoxic, hepatotoxic, immunosuppressive, mutagenic [15], estrogenic and teratogenic effects, depending on exposure levels [16], which are particularly relevant for human consumption of contaminated food [14].

Mycotoxins are secondary fungal metabolites, not essential for the normal growth and reproduction of a fungus, but capable of causing biochemical, physiological, and pathological changes in many species and pose a global threat to public health. Mycotoxins have harmful effects on both humans and animals. These effects include immune toxicity, carcinogenicity, neurotoxicity, teratogenicity, nephrotoxicity, indigestion, hepatotoxicity, developmental and reproductive toxicity, and more. Most mycotoxins can be found in various agricultural products, which are then processed, staple foods and often consumed, which are generally dependent on their composition—food matrix composition, water activity, relative humidity and moisture content of the product, pH, temperature, physical appearance, and degree of damage, as well as the presence of mold spores [17].

Mycotoxins are secondary metabolites toxic to humans and animals [16, 18]. Most of these toxins have relatively low molecular weights and are generally thermally stable demonstrating high levels of bioaccumulation [16, 19]. More than 400 types of mycotoxins have been identified, however, only about 10–15 are considered to be of public health interest [19], with aflatoxin (AF), deoxynivalenol (DON), ergot alkaloids, fumonisins (FB), ochratoxin A (OTA), patulin (PAT), zearalenone (ZEN), and trichothecenes (T-2 and HT-2), the most prominent due to their high incidence in food. OTA and AF can be produced by toxigenic fungi associated with dried meat products [2, 12, 16].

2.1 Aflatoxins (AF)

Aflatoxins (*A-flavus-toxins*) are considered the best known and most toxic mycotoxins. They are produced by certain species of molds of the genus Aspergillus, their growth being thus particularly favored at temperatures between 26°C and 38°C and with a moisture content of more than 18%. Six forms of aflatoxins are identified—aflatoxin B1 (AFB1), aflatoxin B2 (AFB2), aflatoxin G1 (AFG1), aflatoxin G2 (AFG2), aflatoxin M1 (AFM1), and aflatoxin M2 (AFM2). They are reported in several crops, mainly maize, peanuts, pistachios, and cotton seeds. Aspergillus flavus is responsible for the production of aflatoxins B1 and B2, while *Aspergillus parasiticus* can produce aflatoxins B1, B2, G1, and G2, especially in storage time [17, 20, 21].

Aflatoxin B1 (AFB1) is considered the most potent natural carcinogen and is classified by the International Agency for Research on Cancer (IARC) group 1 as carcinogenic to humans. It is estimated that AFB1 causes up to 28% of all liver cancers, and has been associated with impaired immune system growth and dysfunction. AFB1 and its metabolites are excreted in urine, feces, and breast milk [22, 23].

Aflatoxins contamination has been demonstrated in cereals and cereal-based products [24, 25], organs, meat, pork products, and chicken eggs [26, 27]. In addition, aflatoxin M1 is released into milk through the milk glands of cattle fed aflatoxin B1—contaminated feed. Given the stability of the toxin during pasteurization and sterilization of milk and dairy products, even a relatively small amount of aflatoxin M1 can significantly affect human health [28].

2.2 Ochratoxins

The ochratoxin group includes ochratoxins A, B, C, and TA. An ochratoxin molecule is composed of dihydroisocoumarin and the L-β-phenylalanine component. The most toxic representative of the group is ochratoxin A (OTA), isolated from the mold of *Aspergillus ochraceus* [29].

The researchers' reports showed that the genus Penicillium (*P. verrucosum*) and members of Aspergillus (*A. carbonarius* and *A. ochraceus*) are the main producers of the toxin. This toxin can be produced over a wide range of conditions in terms of humidity and temperature, the optimum humidity of crops, for its synthesis, is at least 16%, and the optimum temperatures are between 20 and 25°C [30].

Significant concentrations of ochratoxin A have been found in plant-based foods, such as wheat, corn, rye flower, buckwheat, and breakfast cereals, but the toxin can also be found in offal, meat, and meat products due to secondary contamination [31]. Sources in the literature have reported that the most substantial amounts of ochratoxin A can be found in organ-based meat products [32, 33]. In addition, significant amounts of this mycotoxin have been found in smoked meat products and other animal products [17, 31].

2.3 Zearalenone (ZEN)

The toxin F-2, the mycotoxin zearalenone, received this designation in 1962, after the *Giberella zeae* mold, from which it was isolated. The most important producers of zearalenone are the forms—*Fusarium graminearum, Fusarium culmorum, Fusarium moniliforme, Fusarium roseum, and Fusarium tricinctum* [17].

This mycotoxin is a nonsteroidal estrogen, and its chemical structure is that of resorcylic acid lactone [34]. Zearalenone production is increased especially in wetter, somewhat colder climates, with temperatures of 10–15°C. More than 150 zearalenone derivatives are currently known. The most toxic is considered α-zearalenone. More toxins up to 3–4 times compared to zearalenone. β-Zearalenone is thought to have an activity similar to that of zearalenone. This mycotoxin is thermally stable and stable in several types of solvents, such as ethyl acetate, acetonitrile, acetone, methanol, or chloroform. Zearalenone is insoluble in water but can be dissolved in alkaline water, alcohols, or ether. It is also insoluble in carbon tetrachloride and carbon [17].

Cold wet periods and the early onset of frost, followed by strong periods of sunshine, favor the infestation of crops with Fusarium spp. Before harvest, in this process, zearalenone is also produced [30].

It is commonly found in corn, but can also be found in wheat, barley, sorghum, and rye from countries around the world. Although at much lower concentrations, zearalenone has also been found in milk, meat, organs, and eggs from animals exposed to this mycotoxin through contaminated feed [17].

2.4 Fumonisins (FB)

Fumonisins are the group of mycotoxins produced by molds of the genus Fusarium and comprise fumonisins B1, B2, B3, and B4. The most toxic of these, fumonisin B1, is a propane-1,2,3-tricarboxylic acid diester. Molds that produce fumonisins in significant amounts are *Fusarium verticillioides, Fusarium proliferatum*, and *Fusarium moniliforme*. They are soluble in water, acetonitrile and methanol, thermally stable, and resistant to alkalis that are not photosensitive. The high temperatures used in food processing do not affect their stability.

Substantial amounts of this mycotoxin have been identified in foods intended for the human diet, but also in milk, meat, and eggs of animals feeding on feed contaminated with fumonisin B1, even if they were not found in concentrations harmful to human health. Recently, fumonisins B2 and B4 were produced by *Aspergillus niger* isolated from coffee and fumonisin B2 in *A. niger* from grapes. Fumonisin B2 is detected in coffee beans, wine, and beer [17, 35, 36].

Data from the literature have shown correlations between different diseases such as liver cancer in rats, esophageal cancer in humans, leukoencephalomalacia in horses or donkeys, pulmonary edema in pigs, and contamination with fumonisins. Fumonisin B1, according to IARC, is classified in group 2B as a potential carcinogen for humans [17, 36].

2.5 Deoxynivalenol (DON)

Deoxynivalenol (DON, vomitoxin), is a tetracyclic epoxy sesquiterpene and belongs to the group of trichothecene mycotoxins type B [37] and was first isolated from damaged barley grains in 1972. DON production is mainly attributed to molds *Fusarium gramineraru*m and *Fusarium culmorum* and is enhanced by wetter climates (water activity of 0.97) at temperatures of 25–28°C [17]. DON is a small colorless powder that is soluble in polar solvents, such as water, methanol, ethanol, acetonitrile, and ethyl acetate. It remains stable during storage, grinding, and processing and is, at least to some extent, resistant to heat processing of both food and feed [38].

Among trichothecans, DON is the least toxic, but it is gaining importance due to its high prevalence in food around the globe. The man, who consumes contaminated grains, accuses acute nausea, vomiting, diarrhea, abdominal pain, headache, dizziness, and fever. In animals, acute exposure to DON leads to lower food intake (anorexia) and vomiting, while prolonged exposure may lead to lower yields and thymus, spleen, heart, and liver disease.

The main grains in which DON has been identified are wheat, corn, rye, oats, and barley. They are found, but less often in rice, triticale, or sorghum. Cereals can be contaminated with DON in the field, but also during storage. Consequently, deoxynivalenol can be found in the raw material, the finished food product based on cereals, but also in feed [39]. It has been suggested that DON may also be present in products of animal origin, such as meat and milk [40]. Its metabolites are rapidly excreted from the body, especially in urine, but also in milk, however, in much lower concentrations [17].

2.6 Patulin (PAT)

Molds of the genera *Aspergillus, Byssochlamys*, and *Penicillium* are responsible for the production of the mycotoxin patulin. It can be grown on cereals, fruits, vegetables, processed foods, or on different types of cheese. *Penicillium expansum* is the mold that produces this toxin; it is generally found in the soil and is the most important source of fruit patulin. Patulin, in terms of chemical composition, is a polyketide lactone, made up of a single small molecule. This molecule can be isolated as white or colorless crystals. Patulin is soluble in water, ethanol, methanol, acetone, or ethyl acetate/amyl. Patulin is less soluble in benzene or diethyl ether. This mycotoxin is stable in acidic solutions, but its sulfuric acid can degrade.

Once produced by the mold *Penicillium expansum*, the patulin most often reveals its presence in the form of a disease that affects apples after harvest (rot, rot) or during storage. This mycotoxin has been identified in apples, apple juice, pears, grapes, fodder, and flowers affected by brown rot. Given that consumers, but also producers tend to eliminate the rotten part of fruits or cereals before consumption or processing, the maximum allowed limit for food safety is not exceeded. In the case of cheese, cysteine in high concentrations interacts with patulin and deactivates it. In addition, it has been reported that patulin can be annihilated by fermentation and is, therefore, absent in fruit-based alcoholic beverages and fruit juice-based vinegar, but is present in apple wine (cider). Heat processing manages to moderately reduce the level of patulin; therefore, the patulin found in apple juice maintains its presence during the pasteurization process [17, 41].

2.7 Trichothecenes (T-2 and its main metabolite HT-2)

T-2 toxin together with HT-2, the most important metabolite in or, are produced by molds of the genus Fusarium and are trichothecene type A toxins. This mycotoxin is the basic representative of trichothecine, present in most situations when we talk about trichothecine. It was first identified in maize grown in France. It is a natural sesquiterpene and was isolated from the mold *Fusarium tricinctum*. After several studies, it was concluded that the T-2 toxin can be produced by several species of the genus Fusarium, such as *Fusarium sporotrichioides, Fusarium langsethiae*, and *Fusarium poae*.

The optimal parameters for the development of this mycotoxin are at least 0.88 water activity and a temperature below 15°C, but can be produced between −2°C and 32°C [27, 42]. T-2 toxin is thought to be a powerful cytotoxin and immunosuppressant capable of causing acute intoxication and chronic disease in both humans and animals. Symptoms of acute intoxication include nausea, tremors, abdominal pain, diarrhea, and weight loss [17]. T-2 toxin inhibits protein synthesis, leading to side effects of DNA and RNA synthesis [27]. In addition, it has an adverse effect on the immune system, showing changes in the number of leukocytes and hypersensitivity [42].

Of all cereals, oats are the ones in which contamination with this mycotoxin occurs most frequently and in higher concentrations. Residues and metabolites of T-2 toxin have been found in milk, but not in significantly high concentrations [17, 43].

2.8 Ergot alkaloids

Ergot alkaloids are produced by multiple species of the genus Claviceps. *Claviceps purpurea* is the basic representative of the genus and is the most common in Europe. The most affected cereals are generally rye, wheat, oats, barley, triticale, and millet. Rye is the cereal where this fungus forms sclerotia (dark crescent-shaped bodies that describe the last stage of evolution of plant disease). Pure ergot alkaloids form colorless crystals soluble in organic solvents, such as acetonitrile and methanol, but also in mixtures of organic solvents and buffers. Some of the ergot alkaloids, especially those belonging to the group of simple lysergic acid derivatives, as well as ergoclavins, are soluble in water only to a certain extent. To the extent that more than 50 ergot alkaloids have been isolated from fungal sclerotia, attention has been paid to ergometrine, ergotamine, ergosine, ergocristine, ergocryptine (the latter being a mixture of α- and β-isomers), ergocornine, and their correspondent.

Many mass poisonings caused by the consumption of cereals, flowers, and bread contaminated with ergot alkaloids are recorded throughout human history. If contaminated cereals are consumed in small quantities, one can only expect indigestion, while higher consumption leads to ergotism, that is, the disease that manifests itself with hallucinations, pain, and severe vasoconstriction eventually leading to dry gangrene and numbness of the limbs. The worst-case scenario involves kidney and heart failure and fatal outcomes, while abortion can be induced in pregnant women. A close link between sclerotia content and ergot alkaloid levels has been established in different crops (barley, oats, rye, triticale, and wheat grains) [17, 44].

2.9 Beauvericin—BEA

Beauvericin is a cyclic hexadepsipeptide that is synthesized by various toxigenic fungi, including several species of Fusarium [45]. BEA can be produced by different species of Fusarium in different regions. For example, in the USA and South Africa, *F. circinatum* is the most important BEA-producing fungus, while in Europe, *F. sambucinum* and *F. subglutinans* are the most relevant [46]. As a mycotoxin, BEA is a relevant natural contaminant when referring to mycotoxins in cereals and cereal-based products [47]. BEA contamination is a reported food safety problem in Southern Europe [48]. BEA is toxic to human tissues and cells and has a cytotoxic effect at a lower concentration than that for aflatoxin B1 [49, 50].

2.10 α-Cyclopiazonic acid—CPA

Cyclopiazonic mycotoxin was first discovered in 1968. The species responsible for CPA production are *Aspergillus* (*A. tamarii*, *A. oryzae*, and *A. flavus*) and *Penicillium* (*P. dipodomyicola, P. camemberti, P. griseofulvum,* and *P. commune*). This mycotoxin has been reported in foods such as milk and cheese, oilseeds and nuts, cereals, dried figs, and meat products and has a toxicological effect. It was most commonly detected in products such as peanuts and corn. CPA is toxic to animals such as rats, pigs, guinea pigs, poultry, and dogs. After ingestion of feed contaminated with CPA, the tested animals show severe gastrointestinal disorders and neurological disorders. The affected organs were the liver, kidneys, heart, and digestive tract, which show degenerative changes and necrosis [23].

2.11 Citrinin—CIT

Citrinin is a polyketide mycotoxin, which contaminates food and is associated with various toxic effects. CIT is produced by several fungal strains belonging to the genera *Penicillium, Aspergillus*, and *Monascus* and is usually found together with another nephrotoxic mycotoxin, ochratoxin A. Although, it is clear that exposure to CIT can have toxic effects on the heart, liver, kidneys, and the reproductive system, the mechanism of CIT-induced toxicity remains largely elusive. The presence of CIT has been reported in fruits, fruit juices, beans, vegetables, red rice, herbs, spices, and spoiled dairy products [51].

2.12 Enniatin—ENN

Enniatins are a group of cyclic hexadepsipeptides, comprising 29 enniatin analogs, belonging to groups A and B. Of these analogs, the most commonly found in food (most commonly found in cereals and cereal products) and feed are A, A1, B, B1, although Enniatins B2, B3, and B4 are also found, especially in cereals. This heterogeneous group of mycotoxins is produced by several types of fungi belonging to the genus *Fusarium—F. acuminatum, F. avenaceum, F. oxysporum, F. poae, F. sporotrichioides, F. sambucinum*, and *F. tricinctum* [52, 53].

2.13 Alternaria toxins—ATs

Alternaria is one of the main mycotoxins with a mycotoxigenic effect found in cereals around the world. Although, cereals are constantly affected by Alternaria spp. and their toxins, little relevance is still given to the subject. Currently, tenuazonic acid in sorghum/millet baby foods is the only Alternaria toxin regulated by a government official (the Bavarian Food and Safety Authority) [54].

3. Mycotoxins identified in food

Mycotoxins are not only highly toxic but also widely distributed in various products, such as cereals [55, 56], nuts [57, 58], fruits, vegetables [59], corn [60], seaweed [61], wines [62], meat [12], eggs [63], dried fruits [64], coffee [65], milk [66], and so on. The Food and Agriculture Organization (FAO) has estimated that approximately 25% of world food crops are contaminated with mycotoxins each year [10].

Consumption of foods contaminated with mycotoxins could be the most important source of exposure to toxic mycotoxins, which can be mainly dangerous especially for children and infants [67]. Obviously, a wide mass of mycotoxins can be found in the same product, because a single species of fungus can produce several toxic metabolites, even several species of fungi can be present simultaneously and can produce different toxins [56]. For example, raw cereals are often contaminated with DON and NIV, and other mycotoxins such as AF, ZEN, and OTA are also detected in low-level raw cereals [68]. In addition, DON and ZEN are widespread especially in rice, and mycotoxins such as AF, OTA, and FB1 are also detected in rice [69]. Although mycotoxins are frequently coexisting, different samples may contain only the most common individual mycotoxin. For example, the most common mycotoxin in milk is AFM1, which is also known as "milk toxin." Most investigations are aimed at detecting AFM1 in milk [70]. PAT is usually predominant in fruit-derived products [71]. In addition, the most common mycotoxin in wine is OTA [72]. Migration and environmental accumulation are the other important ways of exposure for people, with the exception of direct input. For example, Schenzel et al. reported that 3-acetyl-deoxynivalenol, DON, NIV, and BEA were detected in Swiss Midland Rivers [73]. A number of researchers have also indicated that drinking water is an important matrix contaminated with mycotoxins [74] and the living environment of humans, these being a principal threat to public health.

The increasing spread of mycotoxins and the highly toxic effects have led to the establishment of organizations that aim to make regulations on the control of food contamination. For example, the FAO a scientific advisory board of the WHO and the Joint Committee of Experts on Food Additives (JECFA) have the responsibility to assess the risks of mycotoxins. In 2001, the Commission's Scientific Committee for Food (SCF) initially set maximum levels for AF, OTA, and PAT in food (EU Regulation 466/2001) (EC, 2001). In addition, the IARC has classified mycotoxins into different categories according to human carcinogenic risk. In addition, the EC has set the maximum levels allowed for most mycotoxins in food by Commission Regulation No. EC 1881/2006, but also methods of sampling and analysis for their control with the help of EC 401/2006 to protect or reduce losses that occur in production and to protect human health. The EC has set maximum limits of 0.012 mg/kg for AFB1 in apricots, pistachios, and almonds; 0.00005 mg/kg for AFM1 in raw or heat-treated milk and dairy products; 0.05 mg/kg for PAT in fruit juices; 0.002 mg/kg for OTA in wine; 0.075 mg/kg for ZEN in cereals; 0.5 mg/kg for DON in bread; 10 mg/kg for the amount of AFG1, AFG2, AFB1, and AFB2 in nuts and peanuts; and maximum limits of 400 μg/kg for ZEN in refined maize germ oil [10].

3.1 Mycotoxins in cereals

Cereals are perhaps the most consumed categories of products worldwide by humans because they are an important source of energy, vitamins, minerals, and fiber [75]. These products can come with different mushrooms from the farm, after harvest, or during storage. Most mycotoxins found in cereals are influenced by poor storage conditions, temperature, climate, drought, or insect damage [76]. The physicochemical composition of cereals, including water activity or pH, can influence the development of mycotoxins [58, 77].

3.2 Mycotoxins in wheat

Wheat contributes to a wide range of bakery products, such as bread, breakfast cereals, biscuits, cakes, pasta, and other cereal-based products. Therefore, the level of contamination of wheat with mycotoxins is essential in the food and feed chain. According to existing studies on wheat seeds, the major occurrence of mycotoxins was DON, ZEN, AFB1, OTA, HT-2/T-2, AF, and FUM, respectively. According to the EC regulation, the recommended limit for wheat mycotoxins is 4 μg/kg for AF, 2 μg/kg for AFB1, 1250 μg/kg for DON, 5 μg/kg for OTA, and 100 μg/kg for ZEN [78].

Of the studies on mycotoxins in wheat grains, 16.6% were reported to exceed EU-recommended limits. The most common were AF with a percentage of 50%, of which 40% were AFB1, followed by ZEN WITH 22.2%. In the case of DON, the highest value, 17,753 μg/kg, was reported in China [79], and in the wheat samples from Qatar Hassan et al. reported DON values of 0.1 μg/kg [78]. For ZEN the highest values were reported in India [80], and the lowest values in Qatar [81]. In the case of AF the highest values, 9 μg/kg, were reported for wheat samples from Qatar [81], the maximum level allowed for the EU being 4 μg/kg, and in wheat samples from Greece AF was not detected [82].

Topi et al. analyzed 10 Fusarium toxins in 71 wheat samples in Albania. The analytical procedure consisted of simple one-step sample extraction, followed by the determination of toxins using liquid chromatography coupled with tandem mass spectrometry. Fusarium toxins were found in 23% of the wheat samples analyzed. In the wheat samples, the only Fusarium mycotoxin detected was deoxynivalenol (DON), present in 23% of the samples, with a concentration of 1916 g/kg, exceeding the maximum level allowed by the EU (1250 g/kg) [83].

According to Malir et al., the most common mycotoxins in wheat flour are aflatoxins B1, B2, G1, G2, ochratoxin A, and deoxynivalenol [84].

3.3 Mycotoxins in corn

Corn seeds are often contaminated with *Fusarium verticillioides* and *Fusarium proliferatum* that produce FUMs toxin. However, other mycotoxins have been found in corn along with FUMs [78]. The highest contamination rate was related to AFB1, ZEN, and DON, respectively. The European Commission (EC) has defined the maximum concentration of mycotoxins in maize. When maize is used for human consumption, these maximum quantities are 4000 μg/kg for FUMs, 1750 μg/kg for DON, 350 μg/kg for ZEN, 5 μg/kg for OTA, 2 μg/kg for AFB1, 10 μg/kg for AFs, and 100 μg/kg for T-2 + HT-2 [10]. In the study conducted by Aristil et al., 87.5% of the samples detected with AFB1, the AF level was higher than the allowed level. This value was 80%, 66.6% for AF and OTA, respectively. For other mycotoxins, the values detected were often lower than the maximum EC values. Existing research has shown that the highest prevalence of AFB1 was in Haiti with 188 44 μg/kg [85], Kenya with 76.2 μg/kg [86], and Serbia with 44 μg/kg [87]. Kos et al. reported a high average prevalence of DON (963 μg/kg), ZEN (163 μg/kg) in Serbia [88]. The high OTA content (1662 μg/kg) is reported in Vietnam [89], and Skendi et al. in Greece reported the lowest OTA levels (0.7 μg/kg) [82]. According to studies by Bertuzzi et al. in Italy [85], the highest FUM content was 43,296 μg/kg [90]. Corn is used as a raw material for flour, breakfast cereals, popcorn, popcorn, and various other foods [78]. Consequently, maize is a good host for mycotoxins, such as AFB1, OTA, ZEN, and DON, and requires continuous monitoring. The presence of these mycotoxins represents a real danger for the entire food chain due to the high consumption of corn [91].

Topi et al. analyzed 10 Fusarium toxins in 45 maize samples from Albania. Fusarium toxins were found in 78% of the maize samples analyzed. In 76% of the corn samples, fumonisins B1 (FB1) and B2 (FB2) were found with concentrations between 59.9 and 16.970 g/kg. The amount of FB1 and FB2 exceeded the maximum level allowed by the EU (4000 g/kg) in 31% of the maize samples [83].

According to Zinedine et al., the most common mycotoxins in cornflakes and corn-based foods are *fumonisins* and *beauvericin* [92].

3.4 Mycotoxins in rice

The mycotoxins identified in rice seeds based on prevalence were AFB1, ZEN, DON, FUM, AF, OTA, and HT-2/T-2 toxins [78].

According to the maximum number of mycotoxins allowed by the EC for rice seeds, the following values are given—4 μg/kg for AF, 2 μg/kg for AFB1, 5 μg/kg for OTA, 100 μg/kg for ZEN, and 1250 μg/kg for DON. Of the studies analyzed, exceedances of the EC standard limit for AF and AFB1 (50%), FUM (25%), DON (16.6%), ZEN (11.1%) were reported. Values exceeding the maximum limits allowed by the EU were also reported in a study conducted in Somalia, where 330 μg/kg AFB1 and 4361 μg/kg FUM were detected in the rice samples [93]. The level of FUM and HT-2/T-2 toxins in all rice samples was below the EU maximum. In China, the maximum allowable level for DON in rice samples is reported at 1607 μg/kg [78].

Several authors have reported that the most common mycotoxins in rice are total aflatoxins, aflatoxin B1, ochratoxin A, and beauvericin [94, 95].

3.5 Mycotoxins in barley, sorghum, oats, and rye

DON was an abundant mycotoxin in barley samples collected from different countries, followed by ZEN and T-2/HT-2 toxins. A study conducted in Canada showed that 56% of cold-season barley presented to the mycotoxin-contaminated industry whose DON concentration in some samples exceeded the regulatory level (1250 μg/kg) [96]. According to several studies conducted in Argentina [97], the Czech Republic [98], and Brazil [99], the main mycotoxin of the genus Fusarium reported in barley samples was DON. In a study conducted in Turkey, in the analyzed barley samples ZEN was not detected, and DON did not exceed the maximum level allowed by the EU (138–973 μg/kg) [100]. DON, FUMs, T-2/HT-2 reported in 50%, 25%, and 50% of barley samples from the Qatar food market with average values of 0.048 mg/kg, 0.553 mg/kg, and 0.067 mg/kg [81].

The most common mycotoxins in sorghum are FUM, AFB1, and ZEN [101]. According to a study conducted in Togo, FUM was detected in 67% of the samples and AFB1 in 25% [102]. In another study conducted in Somalia, the maximum allowable limits for FUM (FB1 and FB2) and AFB1 were exceeded in the sorghum analysis samples [93]. In a study conducted in Tunisia, in the analyzed sorghum samples, the presence of mycotoxins AFB1, OTA, and ZEN was reported, with values between 0.03–31.7 μg/kg, 1.04–27.8 μg/kg, and 3.75–64, 52 μg/kg, respectively [103].

In a study conducted in Nigeria, all sorghum samples analyzed were contaminated with FUM and AF. OTAs have also been identified in some samples [104]. In a study conducted in Switzerland, on oats, by Schöneberg et al., the majority of mycotoxins identified were T-2/HT-2 [105]. In another study conducted in India, the analyzed oat samples were contaminated with ZE in the proportion of 84%, identifying values between 5.31 and 389 μg/kg [80]. In the US study by Jin et al., 75% of the rye samples were contaminated with DON, reporting values below 1.0 mg/kg, but showed an increase through the malting process [106].

According to Meca et al., the most common mycotoxins in barley are deoxynivalenol and beauvericin [107]. The most mycotoxins in cereal porridge are aflatoxins B1, B2, G1, G2 and deoxynivalenol and in breakfast cereals are aflatoxins B1, B2, G1, G2 [108].

3.6 Mycotoxins in fruits, vegetables, and preparations thereof

Fruits and vegetables are extremely sensitive to fungal infestation due to their high water content and abundance of nutrients. They can decompose at any stage of the growth, harvesting, and storage processes, resulting in the production and accumulation of various mycotoxins [109].

Previous work has shown that mycotoxins that contaminate fruits and vegetables mainly include the toxin Alternaria [110], OTA [111], PAT [109, 112], and trichothecenes [113].

Although consumers can cut the rotten parts of fruits and vegetables before consumption, several mycotoxins, especially those mentioned above, may be present in the rest of the parts [113, 114], indicating that the removal of rotten parts cannot completely eliminate mycotoxin contamination.

A study of 20 samples of sweet peppers from two varieties showed that mycotoxins from Fusarium species involved in the internal rot of fruit migrate from contaminated peppers to initially healthy peppers. B fumonisins (1, 2, and 3) and beauvericin were identified after 10 days of incubation in a closed container and 20°C sweet pepper temperature conditions. Fumonisins B (1, 2, and 3) have been identified in lesions and around the tissue, indicating their migration to healthy parts. The values identified were between 690 and 104,000 μg/kg in lesions for fumonisin B (1) and outside the maximum lesion 556 μg/kg. For the other fumonisins, lower values were obtained in the lesions—10,900 μg/kg for fumonisin B (2) and 1287 μg/kg for fumonisin B (3).

In the case of beauvericin, it was identified only in lesions, in a proportion of 95%, with values between 67 and 73,800 μg/kg [114]. A similar study was conducted for the analysis of eight mycotoxins (*Alternaria toxins, ochratoxin A, patulin, and citrinin*) on apple fruits, sweet cherries, tomatoes, and oranges [113].

H. Dong et al. analyzed seven mycotoxins (AOH, AME, TeA, TEN, OTA, PAT, and DON) from cherry tomatoes and two green leafy plants (salad and pakchoi) provided by Food Science and Technology—Guangzhou Harmony, China, and strawberries and tomatoes were bought from the strawberry fields and markets located in Guangzhou, China. All samples were freshly collected and checked for intact and no rotten visible parts. Mycotoxins were not detected in any of the fresh samples. During long storage, TeA was identified for tomatoes and AME and AOH for strawberries. Increased concentrations were observed with storage time. Studies have shown that optimal storage conditions for fresh fruits and vegetables, which include proper packaging and low temperature, help, delay the formation of mycotoxins [59].

Fruits and pomegranate juice from Greek markets were studied by Myresiotis et al. Three Alternaria mycotoxins (alternariol, alternariol monomethyl ether, and tentoxin) were determined, and in fresh samples, they were not identified. However, in the case of artificial inoculation of pomegranate fruits with various species of *Alternaria alternata*, concentrations between 0.3 and 50.5 μg/g were detected, the tentoxin not being detected [111].

A larger study of pomegranate fruits in Greece and Cyprus was presented by Kanetis et al. The fruits were studied before and after harvest. The results show that the rot of pomegranate fruits before harvesting was mainly caused by species of the genera Aspergillus (*Aspergillus niger* and *Aspergillus tubingensis*) and Alternaria (*A. alternata*, *Alternaria tenuissima*, and *Alternaria arborescens*) [115].

And the postharvest fruit spoilage was mainly caused by *Botrytis* spp. and to a lesser extent by isolates of *Pilidiella granati* and *Alternaria spp*. Production of alternariol (AOH), alternative monomethyl ether (AME), and tentoxin (TEN) was estimated among Alternaria isolates, while production of OTA and fumonisin B2 (FB2) was assessed in identified black asparagus. In total, in both countries, 89% of Alternaria isolates produced AOH and AME *in vitro*, while TEN was produced by 43.9%. The data presented imply that the mycotoxin species Alternaria and Aspergillus not only constitute a significant subgroup of the fungal population associated with the rotting of pomegranate fruits responsible for fruit deterioration but also present a potential risk factor for the health of consumers of basic products of pomegranate [115].

Apples, represented by the varieties Fuji, Golden Delicious, Granny Smith, and Red Delicious, in the study conducted by Ntasiou et al. are most affected by mycotoxins—AOH, AME, and TEN [116]. According to Munitz et al. isolated mycotoxins with the potential to be present in blueberries are FB1, FB2, FB3, ZEA, DON, AOH, AME, AFB1, AFB2, AFG1, HT-2, and T-2 [117].

3.7 Mycotoxins in baby food

There is a growing interest in baby food. According to the study conducted by Sarubbi et al., patulin is detected very often in baby food in Italy. According to EC regulation 1881/06, the maximum permitted limit of patulin in baby food is 10 μg/kg or 10 μg/l. A total of 80 homogenized baby foods were analyzed to assess children's exposure to patulin by consuming these products. Experimental tests revealed significant differences between products from organic production and those from traditional production in all categories analyzed. Tomato concentrates showed an average patulin concentration of 7.15 ng/ml of the product; tomato sauce for baby food of 5.23 ng/ml; tomato sauce 4.05 ng/ml; homogenized pear of 0.79 ng/ml, homogenized apple of 0.85 ng/ml. The low incidence of patulin, or low concentrations, in Italian products, is a quality parameter for fruits and their derivatives [112].

The most common mycotoxins in baby food and baby fruits are aflatoxins B1, B2, G1, G2 patulin, and beauvericin [84, 118].

3.8 Mycotoxins in spices

Abrunhosa et al. report the presence in the spice of several mycotoxins such as ochratoxin A, sum of aflatoxin B1, aflatoxin B2, aflatoxin G1, and aflatoxin G2 [119].

3.9 Mycotoxins in wine

Fungal diseases in the vineyard reduce the quality of grapes and affect their volatile profile. Therefore, it influences the taste, aroma, and color of both the juice and the wine. The most common mycotoxins in stubble are aflatoxins, alternariol, OTA, tenuazonic acid, citrinin, patulin, or fumonisin B2.

The countries that provide the most information about wine mycotoxins are the largest wine producers in Europe—France, Italy, and Spain. The most common and worrying mycotoxin in grapes is OTA, produced by Aspergillus carbonarius. The most important factors regarding the determination of the contamination once identified are the climate, the most important factor, and the high temperatures. The highest concentrations of OTA have been identified in southern Europe, where it is warmest. Accurate fungal identification and detection of mycotoxins in fungi are important and practical methods need to be considered. Both white and red wines, dry, sweet, or hardened can be contaminated with mycotoxins. According to reported studies, it seems that OTA appears more often in red and sweet wines, compared to white ones [120].

According to Oteiza et al. mycotoxins such as PAT and OTA were identified in fruit juices and wines collected in Argentina between 2005 and 2013. PATs were identified in 1997 from 5958 samples, with concentrations ranging from 3.0 to 19,622 μg/l, and 510 samples showed PAT levels above 50 μg/l. A total of 1401 with concentrations between 0.15 and 3.6 μg/l. These mycotoxins identified in fruit juices and wines are influenced by fruit type, product type, and year of production [62].

Jesus et al. in their study noticed that the most common mycotoxin in wines in the United States is OTA [121].

3.10 Mycotoxins in beer

Beer is the most consumed alcoholic beverage in the world. Its mycotoxin contamination is a public health concern, especially for heavy drinkers.

Many studies have been published on the fate of mycotoxins in beer production, analyzing the general production process or only part of it and highlighting the physical parameters that lead to variations in mycotoxin concentration [122–124].

Many studies on beer have focused their investigation on DON, which is the most abundant mycotoxin and is the biggest public health problem related to beer consumption [125].

According to EC regulation 1881/2006 and Commission Recommendation, 2013/165/EU, the maximum allowed levels of mycotoxins in the European Union for 13 compounds are regulated. In the case of beer, we refer to cereal products for which the following limits have been established—for AFB1—2 μg/kg, for total AF—4 μg/kg, for ZEN—75 μg/kg, for DON—750 μg/kg, for OTA—5 μg/kg, and for FUMB1 + FUMB2—400 μg/kg. These limits are considered of great importance because beer has high acceptability worldwide, is consumed in large quantities, and avoids the accumulation of mycotoxins, especially for loyal consumers. Mycotoxin contamination can occur at different stages of brewing. Some of them can be transferred from cereals to malt and then to beer due to their high thermal stability (AF, ZEN, and DON) and water solubility of mycotoxins (DON and FUM) [124, 126].

Whatever the origin, numerous surveys on the occurrence of mycotoxins in beer have been conducted worldwide to date, analyzing different styles of brewing. Many surveys of beer are specific to mycotoxin, looking for the appearance and exposure of humans to various Fusarium mycotoxins found in beer. Others are specific to the style of beer, grouping the beer samples according to the production style applied to the malted barley from which they are made [99, 126].

DON and its derivatives, together with AF, FB, ZEA, T-2, and HT-2 are the most studied mycotoxins in beer and barley, respectively. Among the technological processes, the most relevant stages in the beer production process that have an inhibitory effect on mycotoxins are soaking, baking, mixing, fermentation, and clarification. In these stages, mycotoxins are removed with drainage water, used grain and fermentation residues, diluted or destroyed as a result of heat treatment, or adsorbed on the surface.

Germination has no effect on the level of DON in beer but promotes its transformation into its glycosylated derivative (DON-3-Glc). During mixing, enzymes not only stimulate the release of conjugated DON from protein structures but also decrease the initial toxin concentration due to dilution. This step can be a source of contamination with AF and FUM due to corn-free malt adjuvants that are used for the purpose of high levels of fermentable sugars. Even if during cooking there is the possibility of adding to the hop contaminated with mycotoxins, the amount is too small to be significant for the final product. In general, about 60% of ZEN is eliminated with used grains.

To avoid massive economic losses, during the technological process of obtaining beer, various processes are applied to eliminate mycotoxins or prevent contamination with them, such as lactic acid bacteria during malting and beer, ozonation, special yeast strains (known to bind mycotoxins), hot barley grains, water treatment or fungicidal failures in the field [124].

Several authors reported that the most common mycotoxins in malt are aflatoxins B1, B2, G1, G2, OTA, PAT, and DON, and in beer are OTA, DON, and sterigmatocystin [90, 127–129].

3.11 Mycotoxins in coffee, cocoa, and chocolate

According to a meta-analysis by Khaneghah et al. out of 3182 centralized samples from 36 articles, the prevalent and global level of OTA was 53.0% (95% CI: 43.0–62.0) and 3.21 μg/kg (95% CI: 3.08–3.34 μg/kg), respectively. The correlations and the increase of the concentrations of these mycotoxins in the coffee beans were identified, together with the increase of the poverty, but also with the fluctuation of the precipitations from the whole year studied. The lowest concentrations (0.35 μg/kg) of OTA in coffee were reported in Taiwan, and the highest concentrations (79.0 μg/kg) were reported in Turkey [65]. Of the 26 samples of coffee beans and coffee products, 18% were identified with ENN, the average concentration of enniatin was 1901–1901 (g/kg) [130].

According to Batista et al., OTA is the most common mycotoxins in *Arabica coffee* beans [131]. The same mycotoxins are reported in cocoa beans [132].

In a study of chocolate for sale in Brazil, OTA and AF were identified [133]. Similar results were reported by Kabak et al. for chocolate produced in Turkey [134].

3.12 Mycotoxins in water

Several studies report the presence of mycotoxins in portable water, groundwater, and wastewater. The most common are ZEN, aflatoxin B1, B2, G1, and OTA [135–138].

3.13 Mycotoxins in nuts

In the study conducted by Alcántara-Durán et al. on mycotoxins in peanuts, pistachios, and almonds, the lowest concentration level was between 0.05 and 5 μg/kg, being lower than the maximum levels established by current legislation [57].

Another mycotoxin identified in pistachios is aflatoxin B1 (AFB1). Rastegar et al. investigated the effectiveness of the frying process by incorporating lemon juice and/or citric acid on the reduction of AFB1 in contaminated pistachios (AFB1 at two levels of 268 and 383 ng/g). Although frying for 1 hour at 120°C, 50 g of pistachios in 30 ml of lemon juice, 6 g of citric acid, and 30 ml of water, led to a good degradation (93.1%) of AFB1, this treatment changed the desired physical properties. In the case of frying for one hour at 120°C, with 15 ml of lemon juice, 2.25 g of citric acid, and 30 ml of water reduced by 49.2% the level of AFB1, from the initial value, without any visible changes of the pistachio in terms of appearance. Thus, a synergistic effect can be observed regarding the degradation of AFB1 between lemon juice, respectively citric acid and heating. In this situation, we can conclude that in the case of pistachios contaminated with AFB1, they can be degraded by frying with lemon juice and citric acid [58].

According to Abrunhosa et al., the most common mycotoxins in pistachios are aflatoxins B1, B2, G1, G2; in peanuts are aflatoxins B1, B2, G1, G2, OTA, and in almonds are aflatoxins B1, B2, G1, G2 [119].

3.14 Mycotoxins in meat

Consumption of dried meat products is increasing, but these products are highly perishable, and when contaminated with fungi, they pose a risk of human exposure to mycotoxins, and therefore, a global public health problem [139]. Dried meat is composed mostly of muscle tissue in which the physicochemical properties of their surface, such as low water activity, neutral to low pH, and nutrient content, cause the microbial population to grow in external layers of these products [140]. Changes in the low activity of water in these products can influence the metabolism of fungi favoring the biosynthesis of mycotoxins [141].

Xerophilous species of *Aspergillus, Eurotium*, and *Penicillium* have been shown to grow on the surface of dried meat products in different parts of the world, partly due to the tolerance of these microorganisms at low pH and high salt concentrations [142]. Moreover, the maturation time of the product also influences the growth of microorganisms on the surface of these products.

San Daniele ham, for example, contains NaCl concentrations that vary between 10 and 20% of the dry matter and its maturation lasts between 13 and 18 months [14]. Although these salt levels are impossible for many microorganisms to grow, the long maturation period facilitates the growth of microorganisms well adapted to this environment [143]. In addition, abnormal variations in temperature and humidity commonly encountered in the production of traditional products during the pre-ripening, ripening, and drying stages influence the growth of microorganisms [14, 144].

Regarding toxigenic fungi, four aflatoxins, namely B1, B2, G1, and G2, are considered to be some of the most important mycotoxins in dried meat. Aflatoxin B1 is the most common and has a higher toxigenic potential compared to other aflatoxins [12].

In addition to AF, OTA is an important mycotoxin that has been found in dried meat [30]. OTA was first isolated in 1965 from a culture of *Aspergillus ochraceus* [18]. OTA can be transferred from food contaminated with mycotoxin [12].

OTA mycotoxin has been identified in Italian salamis [145] and AFB1 and AFB2 in Egyptian salamis [146]. OTA has also been found in blood sausages, liver-type sausages in Germany [147], Parma ham in Denmark [148], and dried Iberian ham in Spain [144, 149].

In a study in Cairo, burgers and sausages had the highest number of mushrooms compared to fresh meat and canned food. This contamination may be related to the addition of AFB1-contaminated spices to burgers [13].

Among the various forms of direct or indirect human exposure to mycotoxins, such as the intake of contaminated meat products, the relationship with human feed should be considered [12].

In a study of 115 chicken samples collected from central Punjab, Pakistan, the presence of AF, OTA, and ZEN was analyzed. The results showed that 35% of chicken samples were found contaminated with AF, and the maximum level of AFB1 was 7.86 μg/kg and total AF was 8.01 μg/kg found in the hepatic part of the chicken. Furthermore, 41% of chicken samples were found to be contaminated with OTA and a maximum level of 4.70 μg/kg was found in the hepatic part of the chicken meat. A total of 52% of chicken samples were found to be contaminated with ZEN and a maximum level of 5.10 μg/kg. The occurrence and incidence of AF, OTA, and ZEN in chicken meat are alarming and can cause health hazards and have called for the need for continuous monitoring of these toxins in chicken meat [16]. In 70 chicken tissue samples (liver, heart, and pipette) collected from the markets of Jiangsu, Zhejiang, and Shanghai (China) the main mycotoxins observed were DON, 15-AcDON, and ZEN [11].

In a study conducted by Rodrigues, they observed that the most common mycotoxin in Portuguese ham of pork, goat, and sheep is OTA [150].

3.15 Mycotoxins in milk and dairy products

In a study by Ezekiel et al. on mycotoxins in breast milk, complementary foods and urine obtained from 65 infants aged 1–18 months in Ogun State, Nigeria, it was observed that complementary foods were contaminated with six types of mycotoxins, including fumonisins identified in 14 of the 42 samples, with a concentration between 8 and 167 μg/kg and aflatoxins identified in 14 of the 42 samples, with a concentration between 1.0 and 16.2 μg/kg. In four out of 22 breast milk samples, aflatoxin M1 was detected, in addition to six other classes of mycotoxins. And for the first time, dihydrocitrinone was detected in six of the 22 samples studied with a concentration between 14.0 and 59.7 ng/L and sterigmatocystin in a sample of the 22 samples studied with a concentration of 1.2 ng/L. Mycotoxins were detected in 64/65 of urine samples, with seven distinct classes of mycotoxins observed demonstrating ubiquitous exposure. Two metabolites of aflatoxin (AFM1 and AFQ1) and FB1 were detected in samples 6/65, 44/65, and 17/65, respectively. The frequency of detection, the average concentrations, and the appearance of mixtures were usually higher in the urine at nonexclusive breastfeeding, compared to breastfed infants.

In conclusion, the study provides new information on mycotoxin exposure in children in a country at high risk of mycotoxin without adequate food safety measures. Although a small set of samples, it highlights the significant transition to higher levels of mycotoxin exposure in infants as complementary foods are introduced, providing an impetus to alleviate this critical early period and encourage breastfeeding [151, 152].

Other authors also reported the presence of mycotoxins in breast milk such as aflatoxin M1, beauvericin, dihydrocitrinone, alternariol monomethyl ether, enniatin A, enniatin B, ochratoxin A, ochratoxin alpha, ochratoxin B, and sterigmatocystin [153, 154].

In milk powder, the most common mycotoxins reported were aflatoxins B1, B2, G1, G2 [84], in milk aflatoxin M1 [154, 155]. Aflatoxin M1 is also found in cheese [156] or yogurt [119].

Mannami et al. conducted a study on 67 samples of liquid milk (46 pasteurized and 21 UHT) randomly collected during 2019 from supermarkets and dairy stores in four Moroccan cities (Casablanca (n = 27), El Jadida (n = 10), Fez (n = 18), and Meknès (n = 12)). The results showed that out of the 67 samples analyzed, AFM1 was identified in nine samples, while 58 samples (86.6%) had AFM1 below the detection limit. According to Moroccan regulations, the maximum limit allowed by AFM1 is 50 ng/l, and it can be observed that a single pasteurized milk sample exceeds the maximum limit allowed by 77 ng/l, by AFM1. According to Codex Alimentarius standards, where the maximum permitted limit is 500 ng/l, all milk samples studied fall within these limits [157].

A study by Marimón Sibaja et al. carried out between 2003 and 2018 in Latin America on aflatoxin (AFM1) from 3547 milk samples and 969 milk products showed that 67% of milk samples were contaminated with AFM1 and had a concentration between 0.001 and 23.10 μg/kg, and 63% of the dairy samples were contaminated with AFM1 and had a concentration between 0.001 and 18.12 μg/kg. According to these studies, referring to AFM1, the highest estimated daily doses were reported for Mexico (20.9 ng/kg body weight/day), Brazil (2.4 ng/kg body weight/day), Colombia (1.2 ng/kg body weight/day), and Costa Rica (1.0 ng/kg body weight/day). During the 15 years of the study, all average values calculated for Latin American countries exceeded the maximum limits allowed by FAO and WHO (0.058 ng/kg body weight per day) [158].

3.16 Mycotoxins in eggs

In a study of 80 egg samples (farm eggs and domestic eggs) collected from the central areas of Punjab, Pakistan, the presence of AF, OTA, and ZEN was analyzed. The results showed that 28% of the samples were found contaminated with AF, and the maximum level of AFB1 was 2.41 μg/kg and the total AF was 2.97 μg/kg. More than 35% of samples were found to be contaminated with OTA and a maximum level of 1.46 μg/kg. A total of 32% of samples were found to be contaminated with ZEN and a maximum level of 2.23 μg/kg. The occurrence and incidence of AF, OTA, and ZEN in chicken meat are alarming and can cause health hazards and have called for the need for continuous monitoring of these toxins in chicken meat [16].

In 152 egg samples collected from the markets of Jiangsu, Zhejiang, and Shanghai (China) the main mycotoxins observed were DON, 15-AcDON, and ZEN [11]. Makun et al. showed that 85% of eggs tested in Nigeria were contaminated with DON at concentrations between 0.6 and 17.9 ng/g [159].

4. Toxic effects on human health caused by ingestion of mycotoxins

Mycotoxins are a public health concern, mainly due to their multiple types and prevalence that can lead to adverse effects due to chronic exposure even when contaminating food at low levels. If ingested, mycotoxins can cause episodes of acute or chronic diseases, such as various types of cancer, food poisoning, liver disease, various hemorrhagic syndromes, immune and neurological disorders in humans [160]. In addition, mycotoxin contamination of food has been linked to cytotoxicity or even genotoxicity [161], which can also induce toxic effects on the liver and kidneys, immune reproduction and fetal toxicity, and teratogenicity and carcinogenicity [162]. Moreover, exposure to a mycotoxin diet has been associated with an increased incidence of esophageal and gastric carcinomas in certain regions of China [163]. Therefore, mycotoxin contamination is a long-term hidden danger to human health, and relentless efforts have been devoted to mycotoxin investigation [10].

In recent years, large-scale poisoning incidents and international trade disputes caused by fungal contamination are extremely common. For example, severe outbreaks of aflatoxinosis have been reported in Kenya, India, and Malaysia, killing hundreds of people. In the United States, mycotoxin corn infection is a chronic economic and health problem. The European Union's food and feed rapid alert system has placed mycotoxins in second place based on the total number of hazard notifications [10].

Table 1 summarizes the structures of common mycotoxins and the toxic effects they cause on human health. For example, AF toxicity can cause the infant to deform by crossing the placental barrier [183]. In 2018, McMillan et al. confirmed that AF could cause other effects, such as anemia, immunosuppression, and reduced growth rate [165]. In addition, the International Agency for Research on Cancer (IARC) has indicated that exposure to AF may impair renal function in addition to having strong hepatotoxic effects (IARC group 1) (group 1 means carcinogenic to humans), and the same effects have been reported for sterigmatocystin [55]. TA, a toxin produced by *Alternaria alternate*, has been considered the Alternaria mycotoxin with the highest acute toxicity. Referring to human toxicities, TA has been blamed for the onyalai outbreak, a human hematological disease that occurs in Africa [181].

In recent years, large-scale poisoning incidents and international trade disputes caused by fungal contamination are extremely common. For example, severe outbreaks of aflatoxinosis have been reported in Kenya, India, and Malaysia, killing hundreds of people. In the United States, corn mycotoxin infection is a chronic economic and health problem [10]. The European Union's food and feed rapid alert system has placed mycotoxins in second place in terms of the total number of hazard notifications.

CIT affects kidney function but has been shown to be less toxic than OTA. The latter has carcinogenic, neurotoxic, immunotoxic, and teratogenic effects, exerting nephrotoxicity. According to IARC group 2B (group 2B means possible human carcinoma) both OTA and fumonisins have carcinogenic effects on kidney cells) [10]. It is called vomitoxin because it can lead to some typical acute effects, including nausea, vomiting, abdominal pain, diarrhea, headache, dizziness, or fever, which has also been linked to outbreaks of gastroenteritis in animals and humans. In addition, DON acts as a potent inhibitor of protein synthesis and stimulates the pro-inflammatory response, resulting in the impairment of multiple physiological functions. NIV has been demonstrated with immunotoxicity, hematotoxicity, myelotoxicity, and developmental and reproductive toxicity [169]. T-2 is a latent inhibitor of mitochondrial function and protein synthesis. Moreover, T-2 has toxic effects on the skin and mucous membranes [171].

Mycotoxins	Toxic effect	Reference work
Aflatoxin B_1	Development of hepatocellular carcinoma. Cancer and affects the child's development	[164]
	Anemia, immunosuppression, causing reduction growth rate	[165]
Ochratoxin A	Carcinogenic, teratogenic, immunotoxicity, nephrotoxicity, and neurotoxicity	[10, 166]
Zearalenone	Endometrial cancer	[167]
	Disorders of the hormonal balance of the body; prostate, ovarian, cervical, or breast cancers	[168]
Deoxynivalenol	Emesis, anorexia, growth retardation, immunotoxicity, reproduction, and development resulting from maternal toxicity. Altered neuroendocrine signaling, proinflammatory gene induction, disruption of the growth hormone axis, and altered gut integrity	[169]
	Nausea, vomiting, diarrhea, abdominal pain, headache, dizziness, fever, and effects on reproduction	[170]
Fumonisin B_2	Teratogenic, hepatotoxic, and nephrotoxic	[161]
T-2 toxin	A latent inhibitor of mitochondrial function and protein synthesis	[171]
	Causing low growth and side effects on the thymus, spleen, heart, and liver	[172]
Beauvericin	Induction of apoptosis, increases the concentration of cytoplasmic calcium	[173]
Patulin	Impairment of some of the physiological parameters that characterize the intestinal barrier function	[174]
Citrinin	Impaired renal function in addition to strong hepatotoxic effects	[10]
α-Cyclopiazonic acid	Weight loss, nausea, diarrhea, dizziness, muscle necrosis, seizures	[175]
Enniatin B	Cytotoxic effect for different cell lines and reduces the motility of wild boar sperm	[176]
Alternariol	DNA damage	[177]
	Genotoxic in bacteria and mammalian cells *in vitro*	[10]
Sterigmatocystin	Genotoxic cytotoxic effects	[178]
	Induction of DNA damage in HepG2 cells	[179]
Fusaric acid	Modification of neurotransmitter levels by inhibition of dopamine hydroxylase and modulation of tyrosine hydroxylase	[180]
Tenuazonic acid	Inhibition of protein biosynthesis; causing precancerous changes in the esophageal mucosa of mice	[181]
Mycophenolic acid	Nausea, vomiting, stomach cramps, and diarrhea; infections hematological complications (anemia, leukopenia, neutropenia); cytostatic effects on lymphocytes	[182]

Table 1.
Toxic effects caused by the main mycotoxins.

Long-term ingestion of PAT has shown immunotoxicity, mutagenicity, and neurotoxicity in animals [112]. Trichothecenes are a large family of structurally related mycotoxins among which DON is the most common worldwide [184]. DON has high immunotoxic and immunosuppressive effects against a variety of animal and human cells [88].

DAS exerts acute and chronic effects on humans and animals, such as hematotoxicity, growth retardation, lung disorders, immunotoxicity, and cardiovascular effects [26]. In addition, Vidal et al. linked DAS toxicity to distal tubular epithelial necrosis in the kidney [184]. Fumonisins cause a lot of negative effects on humans and animals, such as teratogenic, hepatotoxic and nephrotoxic, esophageal cancer, liver cancer, and neural tube defects [161]. Belhassen et al. confirmed that ZEN stimulates the growth of human breast cancer cells [185], but IARC classified ZEN in group 3 (IARC) (group 3 does not mean carcinogenic effects on humans). In addition, ZEN has strong estrogenic activity and may be an essential etiological agent of infant intoxication, leading to premature enlargement of puberty and breast enlargement. Moreover, IARC reported that FUS-X mainly affects organs that have actively dividing cells, including hematopoietic tissue, spleen, and thymus, as well as exerts intestinal inflammation, inhibits protein synthesis, and induces apoptosis. However, the toxicity of mycotoxins is not stationary, which changes during metabolism in humans and animals [10]. In addition, the assessment of adverse health effects is complicated by multiple exposures to various mycotoxins that can lead to synergistic or antergic toxic effects [186]. Furthermore, the susceptibility of animals and humans varies according to species, age, nutrition, duration of exposure, and other factors [187]. Therefore, the synergistic or antergic toxic effects of different mycotoxins should attract more attention, which is also a new topic in mycotoxin toxicity research.

In addition, a wide range of masked mycotoxins that have been produced by plant phase II metabolism may co-appear as contaminants in addition to parent compounds in food samples. The group of masked mycotoxins comprises both conjugated extractable and related varieties. Bound mycotoxins are attached to carbohydrates or proteins by covalence or non-covalence, which cannot be detected directly and must be released from the matrix by chemical or enzymatic treatment before detection [188]. Regarding the toxicity of masked mycotoxins, on the one hand, these mycotoxins can degrade in free states in the digestive tract of humans and animals, releasing their prototypes of toxins, thus increasing exposure to toxins and posing a greater threat to human health. On the other hand, changes in mycotoxin molecules that reduce or eliminate toxicity can lead to an apparent overestimation of mycotoxin contamination. Thus, it is necessary to understand the fate of masked mycotoxins during food processing and digestion. Khaneghah et al. conducted a comprehensive review of changes in DON masked forms and their occurrence in combination with culmorin in grain-based products [189]. They also comprehensively exposed the characteristics, incidence, control, and fate of DON and its masked forms [190]. However, there are only limited data reported on the occurrence of masked mycotoxins in food, as well as information on the transformation, stability, and release of masked mycotoxins in the food chain. Moreover, masked mycotoxins easily escaped conventional detection due to the biotransformation of their structures, leading to underreporting [191]. In view of the above, it is essential to pay more attention to the subsequent investigation of masked mycotoxins, in particular their occurrence, exposure, toxicity, and nontarget screening.

5. Conclusions

The purpose of this chapter was to analyze the significant types of mycotoxins in food that are consumed directly or indirectly by humans. Studies show that contamination of various mycotoxins is still high in developing countries and remains the main concern in these regions. In recent years, most reports of contamination have been reported for maize, wheat, and rice, respectively. AFB1 are considered the most dangerous mycotoxins and have a high prevalence in cereals that in most studies exceeded the EC permitted limit. DON, ZEN, and FUM are the other significant mycotoxins in cereals, such as barley, sorghum, and oats.

The high stability of mycotoxins during the production, distribution, storage, and processing of cereals was aimed at the contamination of mycotoxins in cereals. Therefore, the development of practical control and management strategies is essential to ensure consumer safety.

Author details

Romina Alina Marc
Faculty of Food Science and Technology, Food Engineering Department, University of Agricultural Sciences and Veterinary Medicine Cluj-Napoca, Cluj-Napoca, Romania

*Address all correspondence to: romina.vlaic@usamvcluj.ro

References

[1] Ayelign A, De Saeger S. Mycotoxins in Ethiopia: Current status, implications to food safety and mitigation strategies. Food Control. 2020;**113**:107163

[2] Udomkun P et al. Mycotoxins in Sub-Saharan Africa: Present situation, socio-economic impact, awareness, and outlook. Food Control. 2017;**72**:110-122

[3] Liu SJ, Wu YN, Chan L. Application of metabonomics approach in food safety research-a review. Food Reviews International. 2020;**36**(6):547-558

[4] Udomkun P et al. Innovative technologies to manage aflatoxins in foods and feeds and the profitability of application—A review. Food Control. 2017;**76**:127-138

[5] Misihairabgwi J et al. Diversity and fate of fungal metabolites during the preparation of oshikundu, a Namibian traditional fermented beverage. World Mycotoxin Journal. 2018;**11**:1-12

[6] Magan N, Aldred D. Post-harvest control strategies: Minimizing mycotoxins in the food chain. International Journal of Food Microbiology. 2007;**119**(1-2):131-139

[7] Paterson RRM, Lima N. How will climate change affect mycotoxins in food? Food Research International. 2010;**43**(7):1902-1914

[8] Wagacha JM, Muthomi JW. Mycotoxin problem in Africa: Current status, implications to food safety and health and possible management strategies. International Journal of Food Microbiology. 2008;**124**(1):1-12

[9] Pandey MK et al. Mitigating aflatoxin contamination in groundnut through a combination of genetic resistance and post-harvest management practices. Toxins. 2019;**11**(6):1-21

[10] Yang Y et al. Recent advances on toxicity and determination methods of mycotoxins in foodstuffs. Trends in Food Science & Technology. 2020;**96**:233-252

[11] Wang L et al. Occurrence and quantitative risk assessment of twelve mycotoxins in eggs and chicken tissues in China. Toxins. 2018;**10**:477

[12] Pizzolato Montanha F et al. Mycotoxins in dry-cured meats: A review. Food and Chemical Toxicology. 2018;**111**:494-502

[13] Darwish WS et al. An overview on mycotoxin contamination of foods in Africa. The Journal of Veterinary Medical Science. 2014;**76**(6):789-797

[14] Comi G, Iacumin L. Ecology of moulds during the pre-ripening and ripening of San Daniele dry cured ham. Food Research International. 2013;**54**(1):1113-1119

[15] Núñez F et al. Selection and evaluation of *Debaryomyces hansenii* isolates as potential bioprotective agents against toxigenic penicillia in dry-fermented sausages. Food Microbiology. 2015;**46**:114-120

[16] Iqbal SZ et al. Natural incidence of aflatoxins, ochratoxin A and zearalenone in chicken meat and eggs. Food Control. 2014;**43**:98-103

[17] Pleadin J, Frece J, Markov K. Chapter Eight—Mycotoxins in food and feed. In: Toldrá F, editor. Advances in Food and Nutrition Research. Cambridge, Massachusetts, United States: Academic Press; 2019. pp. 297-345

[18] Vipotnik Z, Rodríguez A, Rodrigues P. *Aspergillus westerdijkiae* as a major ochratoxin A risk in dry-cured ham based-media. International Journal of Food Microbiology. 2017;**241**:244-251

[19] Turner NW et al. Analytical methods for determination of mycotoxins: An update (2009-2014). Analytica Chimica Acta. 2015;**901**:12-33

[20] Martins C et al. Are data from mycotoxins' urinary biomarkers and food surveys linked? A review underneath risk assessment. Food Reviews International. 2020:1-26

[21] Caceres I et al. Aflatoxin biosynthesis and genetic regulation: A review. Toxins. 2020;**12**(3):1-28

[22] Wu F. Perspective: Time to face the fungal threat. Nature. 2014;**516**(7529):S7

[23] Ostry V et al. Mycotoxins as human carcinogens-the IARC monographs classification. Mycotoxin Research. 2017;**33**(1):65-73

[24] Pleadin J et al. Annual and regional variations of aflatoxin B1 levels seen in grains and feed coming from Croatian dairy farms over a 5-year period. Food Control. 2015;**47**:221-225

[25] Pleadin J et al. Aflatoxin B1 occurrence in maize sampled from Croatian farms and feed factories during 2013. Food Control. 2014;**40**:286-291

[26] Hussain Z et al. Residues of aflatoxin B1 in broiler meat: Effect of age and dietary aflatoxin B1 levels. Food and Chemical Toxicology. 2010;**48**(12):3304-3307

[27] Richard JL. Some major mycotoxins and their mycotoxicoses--an overview. International Journal of Food Microbiology. 2007;**119**(1-2):3-10

[28] Cavaliere C et al. Liquid chromatography/tandem mass spectrometric confirmatory method for determining aflatoxin M1 in cow milk: Comparison between electrospray and atmospheric pressure photoionization sources. Journal of Chromatography. A. 2006;**1101**(1-2):69-78

[29] Battacone G, Nudda A, Pulina G. Effects of ochratoxin a on livestock production. Toxins (Basel). 2010;**2**(7): 1796-1824

[30] Völkel I. The carry-over of mycotoxins in products of animal origin with special regard to its implications for the European Food Safety Legislation. Food and Nutrition Sciences. 2011;**02**:852-867

[31] Pfohl-Leszkowicz A, Manderville RA. Ochratoxin A: An overview on toxicity and carcinogenicity in animals and humans. Molecular Nutrition & Food Research. 2007;**51**(1):61-99

[32] Perši N et al. Ochratoxin A in raw materials and cooked meat products made from OTA-treated pigs. Meat Science. 2014;**96**(1):203-210

[33] Petzinger E, Weidenbach A. Mycotoxins in the food chain: The role of ochratoxins. Livestock Production Science. 2002;**76**(3):245-250

[34] Zöllner P et al. Concentration levels of zearalenone and its metabolites in urine, muscle tissue, and liver samples of pigs fed with mycotoxin-contaminated oats. Journal of Agricultural and Food Chemistry. 2002;**50**(9):2494-2501

[35] Scott PM. Recent research on fumonisins: A review. Food Additives & Contaminants: Part A. 2012;**29**(2):242-248

[36] Wangia-Dixon RN, Nishimwe K. Molecular toxicology and carcinogenesis

of fumonisins: A review. Journal of Environmental Science and Health, Part C. 2021;**39**(1):44-67

[37] Türker L, Gümüş S. A theoretical study on vomitoxin and its tautomers. Journal of Hazardous Materials. 2009;**163**(1):285-294

[38] Rai M, Varma A. Mycotoxins in Food, Feed and Bioweapons. London, New York: Springer Heidelberg Dordrecht; 2010. pp. 1-405

[39] Streit E et al. Current situation of mycotoxin contamination and co-occurrence in animal feed--focus on Europe. Toxins (Basel). 2012;**4**(10):788-809

[40] Cavret S, Lecoeur S. Fusariotoxin transfer in animal. Food and Chemical Toxicology. 2006;**44**(3):444-453

[41] Vidal A et al. The mycotoxin patulin: An updated short review on occurrence, toxicity and analytical challenges. Food and Chemical Toxicology. 2019;**129**:249-256

[42] Creppy EE. Update of survey, regulation and toxic effects of mycotoxins in Europe. Toxicology Letters. 2002;**127**(1-3):19-28

[43] Yang X et al. Review of the reproductive toxicity of T-2 toxin. Journal of Agricultural and Food Chemistry. 2020;**68**(3):727-734

[44] Mulder PP et al. Tropane and ergot alkaloids in grain-based products for infants and young children in the Netherlands in 2011-2014. Food Additives & Contaminants. Part B, Surveillance. 2015;**8**(4):284-290

[45] Tao YW et al. Anticancer activity and mechanism investigation of beauvericin isolated from secondary metabolites of the mangrove endophytic fungi. Anti-Cancer Agents in Medicinal Chemistry. 2015;**15**(2):258-266

[46] Mallebrera B et al. In vitro mechanisms of beauvericin toxicity: A review. Food and Chemical Toxicology. 2018;**111**:537-545

[47] Juan C, Ritieni A, Mañes J. Occurrence of Fusarium mycotoxins in Italian cereal and cereal products from organic farming. Food Chemistry. 2013;**141**(3):1747-1755

[48] Santini A et al. Fusaproliferin, beauvericin and enniatins: Occurrence in food-A review. World Mycotoxin Journal. 2012;**5**:71-81

[49] Wu Q et al. A Review on the synthesis and bioactivity aspects of beauvericin, a fusarium mycotoxin. Frontiers in Pharmacology. 2018; **9**(1338)

[50] Svingen T et al. Enniatin B and beauvericin are common in Danish cereals and show high hepatotoxicity on a high-content imaging platform. Environmental Toxicology. 2017;**32**(5): 1658-1664

[51] de Oliveira Filho JWG et al. A comprehensive review on biological properties of citrinin. Food and Chemical Toxicology. 2017;**110**:130-141

[52] Fraeyman S et al. Emerging *Fusarium* and *Alternaria* mycotoxins: Occurrence, toxicity and toxicokinetics. Toxins (Basel). 2017;**9**(7):1-30

[53] Prosperini A et al. A review of the mycotoxin enniatin B. Frontiers in Public Health. 2017;**5**:304

[54] Tralamazza SM et al. Toxigenic Alternaria species: Impact in cereals worldwide. Current Opinion in Food Science. 2018;**23**:57-63

[55] Mousavi Khaneghah A et al. Prevalence and concentration of ochratoxin A, zearalenone, deoxynivalenol and total aflatoxin in cereal-based products: A systematic review and meta-analysis. Food and Chemical Toxicology. 2018;**118**:830-848

[56] Mousavi Khaneghah A et al. Aflatoxins in cereals: State of the art. Journal of Food Safety. 2018;**38**(6):e12532

[57] Alcántara-Durán J et al. Use of a modified QuEChERS method for the determination of mycotoxin residues in edible nuts by nano flow liquid chromatography high resolution mass spectrometry. Food Chemistry. 2019;**279**:144-149

[58] Rastegar H et al. Removal of aflatoxin B1 by roasting with lemon juice and/or citric acid in contaminated pistachio nuts. Food Control. 2017;**71**:279-284

[59] Dong H et al. Development and comparison of single-step solid phase extraction and QuEChERS clean-up for the analysis of 7 mycotoxins in fruits and vegetables during storage by UHPLC-MS/MS. Food Chemistry. 2019;**274**:471-479

[60] Dong M et al. Multi-walled carbon nanotubes as solid-phase extraction sorbents for simultaneous determination of type A trichothecenes in maize, wheat and rice by ultra-high performance liquid chromatography-tandem mass spectrometry. Journal of Chromatography A. 2015;**1423**:177-182

[61] Gillibert R, Triba MN, de la Chapelle ML. Surface enhanced Raman scattering sensor for highly sensitive and selective detection of ochratoxin A. Analyst. 2018;**143**(1):339-345

[62] Oteiza JM et al. Influence of production on the presence of patulin and ochratoxin A in fruit juices and wines of Argentina. LWT. 2017;**80**:200-207

[63] Xu X et al. Development of a modified QuEChERS method based on magnetic multiwalled carbon nanotubes for the simultaneous determination of veterinary drugs, pesticides and mycotoxins in eggs by UPLC-MS/MS. Food Chemistry. 2019;**276**:419-426

[64] Heshmati A et al. Co-occurrence of aflatoxins and ochratoxin A in dried fruits in Iran: Dietary exposure risk assessment. Food and Chemical Toxicology. 2017;**106**(Pt A):202-208

[65] Khaneghah AM et al. The concentration and prevalence of ochratoxin A in coffee and coffee-based products: A global systematic review, meta-analysis and meta-regression. Fungal Biology. 2019;**123**(8):611-617

[66] Sengling Cebin Coppa CF et al. The occurrence of mycotoxins in breast milk, fruit products and cereal-based infant formula: A review. Trends in Food Science & Technology. 2019;**92**:81-93

[67] Khlangwiset P, Shephard GS, Wu F. Aflatoxins and growth impairment: A review. Critical Reviews in Toxicology. 2011;**41**(9):740-755

[68] Soleimany F, Jinap S, Abas F. Determination of mycotoxins in cereals by liquid chromatography tandem mass spectrometry. Food Chemistry. 2012;**130**(4):1055-1060

[69] da Silva LP et al. Development and validation of a multianalyte method for quantification of mycotoxins and pesticides in rice using a simple dilute and shoot procedure and UHPLC-MS/MS. Food Chemistry. 2019;**270**:420-427

[70] Rahmani J et al. The prevalence of aflatoxin M1 in milk of Middle

East region: A systematic review, meta-analysis and probabilistic health risk assessment. Food and Chemical Toxicology. 2018;**118**:653-666

[71] Sadok I, Szmagara A, Staniszewska MM. The validated and sensitive HPLC-DAD method for determination of patulin in strawberries. Food Chemistry. 2018;**245**:364-370

[72] Andrade MA, Lanças FM. Determination of Ochratoxin A in wine by packed in-tube solid phase microextraction followed by high performance liquid chromatography coupled to tandem mass spectrometry. Journal of Chromatography. A. 2017;**1493**:41-48

[73] Schenzel J et al. Mycotoxins in the environment: I. Production and emission from an agricultural test field. Environmental Science & Technology. 2012;**46**(24):13067-13075

[74] Emídio ES, da Silva CP, de Marchi MR. Determination of estrogenic mycotoxins in environmental water samples by low-toxicity dispersive liquid-liquid microextraction and liquid chromatography-tandem mass spectrometry. Journal of Chromatography. A. 2015;**1391**:1-8

[75] Pereira VL, Fernandes JO, Cunha SC. Mycotoxins in cereals and related foodstuffs: A review on occurrence and recent methods of analysis. Trends in Food Science & Technology. 2014;**36**(2):96-136

[76] Vasseghian Y et al. A review on mycotoxins detection techniques in edible oils. International Journal of Environmental Analytical Chemistry. 2020

[77] Mousavi Khaneghah A et al. Mycotoxins in cereal-based products during 24 years (1983-2017): A global systematic review. Trends in Food Science & Technology. 2019;**91**:95-105

[78] Khodaei D, Javanmardi F, Khaneghah AM. The global overview of the occurrence of mycotoxins in cereals: A three-year survey. Current Opinion in Food Science. 2021;**39**:36-42

[79] Xu W, Han X, Li F. Co-occurrence of multi-mycotoxins in wheat grains harvested in Anhui province, China. Food Control. 2019;**96**:180-185

[80] Rai A et al. Presence of zearalenone in cereal grains and its exposure risk assessment in Indian population. Journal of Food Science. 2018;**83**(12): 3126-3133

[81] Hassan ZU et al. Prevalence of Fusarium fungi and their toxins in marketed feed. Food Control. 2019;**104**:224-230

[82] Skendi A et al. Presence of mycotoxins, heavy metals and nitrate residues in organic commercial cereal-based foods sold in the Greek market. Journal of Consumer Protection and Food Safety. 2020;**15**(2):109-119

[83] Topi D et al. Incidence of *Fusarium* mycotoxins in wheat and maize from Albania. Molecules. 2021;**26**(1):1-14

[84] Malir F et al. Monitoring the mycotoxins in food and their biomarkers in the Czech Republic. Molecular Nutrition & Food Research. 2006;**50**(6):513-518

[85] Aristil J et al. Fungal contamination and aflatoxin content of maize, moringa and peanut foods from rural subsistence farms in South Haiti. Journal of Stored Products Research. 2020;**85**:101550

[86] Nabwire WR et al. Aflatoxin in household maize for human consumption in Kenya, East Africa. Food Additives & Contaminants: Part B. 2020;**13**(1):45-51

[87] Janić Hajnal E et al. Mycotoxins in maize harvested in Serbia in the period 2012-2015. Part 2: Non-regulated mycotoxins and other fungal metabolites. Food Chemistry. 2020;**317**:126409

[88] Kos J et al. The influence of climate conditions on the occurrence of deoxynivalenol in maize harvested in Serbia during 2013-2015. Food Control. 2017;**73**:734-740

[89] Do TH et al. Dietary exposure and health risk characterization of aflatoxin B1, ochratoxin A, fumonisin B1, and zearalenone in food from different provinces in Northern Vietnam. Food Control. 2020;**112**:107108

[90] Bertuzzi T et al. Co-occurrence of moniliformin and regulated *Fusarium* toxins in maize and wheat grown in Italy. Molecules. 2020;**25**(10):1-13

[91] Škrbić B et al. Levels of aflatoxin M1 in different types of milk collected in Serbia: Assessment of human and animal exposure. Food Control. 2014;**40**:113-119

[92] Zinedine A et al. Further data on the occurrence of Fusarium emerging mycotoxins enniatins (A, A1, B, B1), fusaproliferin and beauvericin in raw cereals commercialized in Morocco. Food Control. 2011;**22**(1):1-5

[93] Wielogorska E et al. Occurrence and human-health impacts of mycotoxins in Somalia. Journal of Agricultural and Food Chemistry. 2019;**67**(7):2052-2060

[94] Toman J et al. The occurrence of ochratoxin A in white and parboiled rice. Czech Journal of Food Sciences. 2016;**34**:32-38

[95] Sifou A et al. First report on the presence of emerging Fusarium mycotoxins enniatins (A, A1, B, B1), beauvericin and fusaproliferin in rice on the Moroccan retail markets. Food Control. 2011;**22**(12):1826-1830

[96] Shi H, Schwab W, Yu P. Natural occurrence and co-contamination of twelve mycotoxins in industry-submitted cool-season cereal grains grown under a low heat unit climate condition. Toxins. 2019;**11**(3):1-9

[97] Nogueira MS et al. Natural contamination with mycotoxins produced by *Fusarium graminearum* and *Fusarium poae* in malting barley in Argentina. Toxins (Basel). 2018;**10**(2):1-13

[98] Svoboda Z et al. The occurrence of the selected Fusarium mycotoxins in Czech malting barley, harvested in 2012-2017. Czech Journal of Food Sciences. 2019;**37**:439-445

[99] Piacentini KC et al. Occurrence of deoxynivalenol and zearalenone in brewing barley grains from Brazil. Mycotoxin Research. 2018;**34**(3):173-178

[100] Golge O, Kabak B. Occurrence of deoxynivalenol and zearalenone in cereals and cereal products from Turkey. Food Control. 2020;**110**:106982

[101] Neme K, Mohammed A. Mycotoxin occurrence in grains and the role of postharvest management as a mitigation strategies. A review. Food Control. 2017;**78**:412-425

[102] Hanvi DM et al. Natural occurrence of mycotoxins in maize and sorghum in Togo. Mycotoxin Research. 2019;**35**(4):321-327

[103] Lahouar A et al. Aflatoxin B1, ochratoxin A and zearalenone in sorghum grains marketed in Tunisia. Food Additives & Contaminants: Part B. 2018;**11**(2):103-110

[104] Onyedum SC et al. Occurrence of major mycotoxins and their dietary

exposure in North-Central Nigeria staples. Scientific African. 2020;**7**:e00188

[105] Schöneberg T et al. Occurrence of Fusarium species and mycotoxins in Swiss oats—Impact of cropping factors. European Journal of Agronomy. 2018;**92**:123-132

[106] Jin Z et al. Malting of fusarium head blight-infected rye (*Secale cereale*): Growth of *Fusarium graminearum*, trichothecene production, and the impact on malt quality. Toxins. 2018;**10**(9):1-15

[107] Meca G et al. Further data on the presence of Fusarium emerging mycotoxins enniatins, fusaproliferin and beauvericin in cereals available on the Spanish markets. Food and Chemical Toxicology. 2010;**48**(5):1412-1416

[108] Martins C et al. Assessment of multiple mycotoxins in breakfast cereals available in the Portuguese market. Food Chemistry. 2018;**239**:132-140

[109] Zia-Ul-Haq M. Past, present and future of carotenoids research. In: Carotenoids: Structure and Function in the Human Body. New York: Springer; 2021

[110] De Berardis S et al. Determination of four *Alternaria alternata* mycotoxins by QuEChERS approach coupled with liquid chromatography-tandem mass spectrometry in tomato-based and fruit-based products. Food Research International. 2018;**106**:677-685

[111] Myresiotis CK et al. Determination of mycotoxins in pomegranate fruits and juices using a QuEChERS-based method. Food Chemistry. 2015;**182**:81-88

[112] Sarubbi F et al. Patulin in homogenized fruit's and tomato products. Food Control. 2016;**59**: 420-423

[113] Wang M et al. A single-step solid phase extraction for the simultaneous determination of 8 mycotoxins in fruits by ultra-high performance liquid chromatography tandem mass spectrometry. Journal of Chromatography A. 2016;**1429**:22-29

[114] Monbaliu S et al. Production and migration of mycotoxins in sweet pepper analyzed by multimycotoxin LC-MS/MS. Journal of Agricultural and Food Chemistry. 2010;**58**(19):10475-10479

[115] Kanetis L et al. Identification and mycotoxigenic capacity of fungi associated with pre- and postharvest fruit rots of pomegranates in Greece and Cyprus. International Journal of Food Microbiology. 2015;**208**:84-92

[116] Ntasiou P et al. Identification, characterization and mycotoxigenic ability of Alternaria spp. causing core rot of apple fruit in Greece. International Journal of Food Microbiology. 2015;**197**:22-29

[117] Munitz MS et al. Mycotoxigenic potential of fungi isolated from freshly harvested Argentinean blueberries. Mycotoxin Research. 2014;**30**(4):221-229

[118] Mahnine N et al. Further data on the levels of emerging Fusarium mycotoxins enniatins (A, A1, B, B1), beauvericin and fusaproliferin in breakfast and infant cereals from Morocco. Food Chemistry. 2011;**124**(2):481-485

[119] Abrunhosa L et al. A review of mycotoxins in food and feed products in Portugal and estimation of probable daily intakes. Critical Reviews in Food Science and Nutrition. 2016;**56**(2):249-265

[120] Paterson RRM et al. Predominant mycotoxins, mycotoxigenic fungi and climate change related to wine. Food Research International. 2018;**103**: 478-491

[121] De Jesus CL et al. High incidence and levels of ochratoxin A in wines sourced from the United States. Toxins. 2018;**10**(1)

[122] Inoue T et al. Fate of mycotoxins during beer brewing and fermentation. Bioscience, Biotechnology, and Biochemistry. 2013;**77**(7):1410-1415

[123] Vaclavikova M et al. 'Emerging' mycotoxins in cereals processing chains: Changes of enniatins during beer and bread making. Food Chemistry. 2013;**136**(2):750-757

[124] Pascari X et al. Mycotoxins and beer. Impact of beer production process on mycotoxin contamination. A review. Food Research International. 2018;**103**:121-129

[125] Kuzdraliński A, Solarska E, Muszyńska M. Deoxynivalenol and zearalenone occurence in beers analysed by an enzyme-linked immunosorbent assay method. Food Control. 2013;**29**(1): 22-24

[126] Rodríguez-Carrasco Y et al. Occurrence of Fusarium mycotoxins and their dietary intake through beer consumption by the European population. Food Chemistry. 2015;**178**:149-155

[127] Mastanjević K et al. Malting and brewing industries encounter Fusarium spp. related problems. Fermentation. 2018;**4**:3

[128] Mastanjević K et al. From malt to wheat beer: A comprehensive multi-toxin screening, transfer assessment and its influence on basic fermentation parameters. Food Chemistry. 2018;**254**:115-121

[129] Peters J et al. Mycotoxin profiling of 1000 beer samples with a special focus on craft beer. PLoS One. 2017;**12**(10):e0185887

[130] Filippo R, Gallo A, Terenzio B. Emerging mycotoxins in the food chain. Mediterranean Journal of Nutrition and Metabolism. 2020;**13**:1-21

[131] Batista LR et al. Ochratoxin A in coffee beans (*Coffea arabica* L.) processed by dry and wet methods. Food Control. 2009;**20**(9):784-790

[132] Raters M, Matissek R. Study on distribution of mycotoxins in cocoa beans. Mycotoxin Research. 2005;**21**:182-186

[133] Copetti MV et al. Co-occurrence of ochratoxin a and aflatoxins in chocolate marketed in Brazil. Food Control. 2012;**26**(1):36-41

[134] Kabak B. Prevention and Management of Mycotoxins in Food and Feed. Berlin, Heidelberg: Springer-Verlag; 2010. pp. 201-227

[135] Paterson R. Zearalenone production and growth in drinking water inoculated with *Fusarium graminearum* (Erratum). Mycological Progress. 2007;**6**:115

[136] Gromadzka K et al. Occurrence of estrogenic mycotoxin—zearalenone in aqueous environmental samples with various NOM content. Water Research. 2009;**43**(4):1051-1059

[137] Hartmann N et al. Quantification of estrogenic mycotoxins at the ng/L level in aqueous environmental samples using deuterated internal standards. Journal of Chromatography A. 2007;**1138**(1):132-140

[138] Mata AT et al. Bottled water: Analysis of mycotoxins by LC-MS/MS. Food Chemistry. 2015;**176**:455-464

[139] Martins FA et al. Daily intake estimates of fumonisins in corn-based food products in the population of Parana, Brazil. Food Control. 2012;**26**(2):614-618

[140] Simoncini N et al. Effect of added autochthonous yeasts on the volatile compounds of dry-cured hams. International Journal of Food Microbiology. 2015;**212**:25-33

[141] Rodríguez A et al. Evaluation of hazard of aflatoxin B1, ochratoxin A and patulin production in dry-cured ham and early detection of producing moulds by qPCR. Food Control. 2012;**27**(1):118-126

[142] Plavsic D et al. Microbiological and chemical evaluation of dried smoked meat product. Procedia Food Science. 2015;**5**:239-242

[143] Rodríguez A et al. The influence of salt (NaCl) on ochratoxin A biosynthetic genes, growth and ochratoxin A production by three strains of *Penicillium nordicum* on a dry-cured ham-based medium. International Journal of Food Microbiology. 2014;**178**:113-119

[144] Rodríguez A et al. Presence of ochratoxin A on the surface of dry-cured Iberian ham after initial fungal growth in the drying stage. Meat Science. 2012;**92**(4):728-734

[145] Iacumin L et al. Moulds and ochratoxin A on surfaces of artisanal and industrial dry sausages. Food Microbiology. 2009;**26**(1):65-70

[146] Aziz NH, Youssef YA. Occurrence of aflatoxins and aflatoxin-producing moulds in fresh and processed meat in Egypt. Food Additives & Contaminants. 1991;**8**(3):321-331

[147] Gareis M, Scheuer R. Ochratoxin A in meat and meat products. Archiv für Lebensmittelhygiene. 2000;**51**(4/5):102-104

[148] Sørensen LM, Mogensen J, Nielsen KF. Simultaneous determination of ochratoxin A, mycophenolic acid and fumonisin B(2) in meat products. Analytical and Bioanalytical Chemistry. 2010;**398**(3):1535-1542

[149] Rodríguez A et al. Effect of selected protective cultures on ochratoxin A accumulation in dry-cured Iberian ham during its ripening process. LWT—Food Science and Technology. 2015;**60**(2, Part 1):923-928

[150] Rodrigues P et al. Mycobiota and mycotoxins in Portuguese pork, goat and sheep dry-cured hams. Mycotoxin Research. 2019;**35**:1-8

[151] Akinyemi M et al. A review of microbes and chemical contaminants in dairy products in sub-Saharan Africa. Comprehensive Reviews in Food Science and Food Safety. 2021

[152] Ezekiel C, Ortega-Beltran A, Bandyopadhyay R. The Need for Integrated Approaches to Address Food Safety Risk: The Case of Mycotoxins in Africa. 2019

[153] Muñoz K et al. Exposure of infants to ochratoxin A with breast milk. Archives of Toxicology. 2014;**88**(3):837-846

[154] Muñoz K et al. Exposure of neonates to ochratoxin A: First biomonitoring results in human milk (colostrum) from Chile. Mycotoxin Research. 2010;**26**(2):59-67

[155] Duarte SC et al. Aflatoxin M1 in marketed milk in Portugal: Assessment of human and animal exposure. Food Control. 2013;**30**(2):411-417

[156] Martins H et al. Aflatoxin M1 determination in cheese by immunoaffinity column clean-up coupled to high-performance liquid chromatography. Revista Portuguesa de Ciências Veterinárias. 2007;**102**:321-325

[157] Mannani N et al. Aflatoxin M1 in pasteurized and UHT milk marked in Morocco. Food Control. 2021;**124**:107893

[158] Marimón Sibaja KV et al. Dietary exposure assessment of aflatoxin M1 in milk and dairy products of Latin America. Food Reviews International. 2021:1-14

[159] Makun H et al. Fungal and aflatoxin contamination of some human food commodities in Nigeria. African Journal of Food Science. 2010;**4**:127-135

[160] Capriotti AL et al. Multiclass mycotoxin analysis in food, environmental and biological matrices with chromatography/mass spectrometry. Mass Spectrometry Reviews. 2012;**31**(4):466-503

[161] Alshannaq A, Yu J-H. Occurrence, toxicity, and analysis of major mycotoxins in food. International Journal of Environmental Research and Public Health. 2017;**14**(6):1-20

[162] Chen C, Wu F. The need to revisit ochratoxin A risk in light of diabetes, obesity, and chronic kidney disease prevalence. Food and Chemical Toxicology. 2017;**103**:79-85

[163] Hsia CC et al. Nivalenol, a main Fusarium toxin in dietary foods from high-risk areas of cancer of esophagus and gastric cardia in China, induced benign and malignant tumors in mice. Oncology Reports. 2004;**12**(2):449-456

[164] Rushing BR, Selim MI. Aflatoxin B1: A review on metabolism, toxicity, occurrence in food, occupational exposure, and detoxification methods. Food and Chemical Toxicology. 2019;**124**: 81-100

[165] McMillan A et al. Aflatoxin exposure in Nigerian children with severe acute malnutrition. Food and Chemical Toxicology. 2018;**111**:356-362

[166] Bui-Klimke TR, Wu F. Ochratoxin A and human health risk: A review of the evidence. Critical Reviews in Food Science and Nutrition. 2015;**55**(13):1860-1869

[167] Pajewska M et al. The determination of zearalenone and its major metabolites in endometrial cancer tissues. Analytical and Bioanalytical Chemistry. 2018;**410**(5):1571-1582

[168] Rogowska A et al. Zearalenone and its metabolites: Effect on human health, metabolism and neutralisation methods. Toxicon. 2019;**162**:46-56

[169] Pestka JJ. Deoxynivalenol: Mechanisms of action, human exposure, and toxicological relevance. Archives of Toxicology. 2010;**84**(9):663-679

[170] Sobrova P et al. Deoxynivalenol and its toxicity. Interdisciplinary Toxicology. 2010;**3**:94-99

[171] Gohar UF, Iqbal I, Shah Z, Mukhtar H, Zia-Ul-Haq M. COVID-19: Recent developments in therapeutic approaches. In: Zia-Ul-Haq M, Bin-Jumah MN, Alothamn SI, Henidi HA, editors. Alternative Medicine Interventions for COVID-19. Vol. 2021. Cham, Switzerland: Springer. pp. 249-274

[172] Aupanun S et al. An overview of the toxicology and toxicokinetics of fusarenon-X, a type B trichothecene mycotoxin. The Journal of Veterinary Medical Science. 2017;**79**(1):6-13

[173] Luz C et al. Occurrence, toxicity, bioaccessibility and mitigation strategies of beauvericin, a minor Fusarium mycotoxin. Food and Chemical Toxicology. 2017;**107**(Pt A):430-439

[174] Akbari P et al. The intestinal barrier as an emerging target in the toxicological assessment of mycotoxins. Archives of Toxicology. 2017;**91**(3):1007-1029

[175] Heperkan D et al. Natural contamination of cyclopiazonic acid in

dried figs and co-occurrence of aflatoxin. Food Control. 2012;**23**(1):82-86

[176] Wätjen W et al. Enniatins A1, B and B1 from an endophytic strain of *Fusarium tricinctum* induce apoptotic cell death in H4IIE hepatoma cells accompanied by inhibition of ERK phosphorylation. Molecular Nutrition & Food Research. 2009;**53**(4):431-440

[177] Solhaug A, Eriksen GS, Holme JA. Mechanisms of action and toxicity of the mycotoxin alternariol: A review. Basic & Clinical Pharmacology & Toxicology. 2016;**119**(6):533-539

[178] Zouaoui N et al. Cytotoxic effects induced by patulin, sterigmatocystin and beauvericin on CHO-K1 cells. Food and Chemical Toxicology. 2016;**89**:92-103

[179] Gao W et al. Sterigmatocystin-induced oxidative DNA damage in human liver-derived cell line through lysosomal damage. Toxicology In Vitro. 2015;**29**(1):1-7

[180] Appell M et al. Determination of fusaric acid in maize using molecularly imprinted SPE clean-up. Journal of Separation Science. 2014;**37**(3):281-286

[181] Yekeler H et al. Analysis of toxic effects of Alternaria toxins on esophagus of mice by light and electron microscopy. Toxicologic Pathology. 2001;**29**(4):492-497

[182] Kiang TKL, Ensom MHH. Exposure-toxicity relationships of mycophenolic acid in adult kidney transplant patients. Clinical Pharmacokinetics. 2019;**58**(12): 1533-1552

[183] Abdulrazzaq YM, Osman N, Ibrahim A. Fetal exposure to aflatoxins in the United Arab Emirates. Annals of Tropical Paediatrics. 2002;**22**(1):3-9

[184] Vidal A et al. Mycotoxin biomarkers of exposure: A comprehensive review. Comprehensive Reviews in Food Science and Food Safety. 2018;**17**(5):1127-1155

[185] Belhassen H et al. Zearalenone and its metabolites in urine and breast cancer risk: A case-control study in Tunisia. Chemosphere. 2015;**128**:1-6

[186] Ficheux AS, Sibiril Y, Parent-Massin D. Co-exposure of Fusarium mycotoxins: In vitro myelotoxicity assessment on human hematopoietic progenitors. Toxicon. 2012;**60**(6):1171-1179

[187] Cigić IK, Prosen H. An overview of conventional and emerging analytical methods for the determination of mycotoxins. International Journal of Molecular Sciences. 2009;**10**(1):62-115

[188] Berthiller F et al. Masked mycotoxins: A review. Molecular Nutrition & Food Research. 2013;**57**(1):165-186

[189] Mousavi Khaneghah A et al. Changes in masked forms of deoxynivalenol and their co-occurrence with culmorin in cereal-based products: A systematic review and meta-analysis. Food Chemistry. 2019;**294**:587-596

[190] Khaneghah AM et al. Deoxynivalenol and its masked forms: Characteristics, incidence, control and fate during wheat and wheat based products processing—A review. Trends in Food Science & Technology. 2018;**71**:13-24

[191] Stoev SD. Foodborne mycotoxicoses, risk assessment and underestimated hazard of masked mycotoxins and joint mycotoxin effects or interaction. Environmental Toxicology and Pharmacology. 2015;**39**(2):794-809

Section 2

The Influence of Contaminants on Food Safety

Chapter 2

The Influence of Some Contaminants in Food Quality

Marisa Nicolai, Paula Pereira and Lídia Palma

Abstract

The concept of food quality has been following scientific and technological evolution. Currently, producers, users, consumers, as well as public authorities, have well defined their expectations regarding the quality requirements in the food sector. These projections are related to several parameters that are no longer seen only from a safety and nutritional point of view. Thus, the characteristics of food products must fulfill criteria that embrace their origin, esthetics, convenience, functionality, ethics, organoleptic and must result in benefit. The needs of consumers increasingly reflect public interests, which are supervised by public authorities that hold technical and scientific information that allows them to advocate normative regulations regarding defects, adulteration, and fraud, increasing awareness in the food quality field. Since food quality and safety are two increasingly interconnected domains, the different EU legislation and regulations impose procedures for the determination of contaminants. In this chapter, we will only cover three main topics, namely heavy metals, polycyclic aromatic hydrocarbons, and mycotoxins.

Keywords: food quality, safety, polycyclic aromatic hydrocarbons, heavy metals, mycotoxins

1. Introduction

Food quality is a very broad concept, whose definition presents a complex and dynamic character, which varies according to the time interval and the geographic location.

From the consumer's point of view, quality is intrinsically linked to health, well-being, and sensory aspect of the products, which makes this concept quite diffuse and subjective [1, 2].

The measurability of the food quality parameter can allow its conversion to be more objective. For producers, the precision in the parameterization of this concept is very important, because the consumer's perception of quality greatly affects the purchase decision, which in Europe is directly correlated with information subjective [2].

According to Tothill and Stephen [3], a large investment is needed in terms of providing relevant information and industrial marketing practices. This gap has been reduced with the regulation on labeling, requiring the definition of consistent norms and standards, a rigorous food quality control process in order to keep the consumer safe [4], and confident in their decision to purchase the product. This point is in line with Organization for Economic Co-operation and Development (OECD) indications, as there are data indicating that the content of food labels influences consumer behavior more than energy efficiency labeling [5].

Food quality control involves the specification of ingredients and the consequent physical, chemical, and microbiological characterization of food and food products [6].

All food quality control is carried out, using acceptable and well-established methodologies, in order to maintain product characteristics, but is increasingly associated with food safety, for the prevention of chemical and biological hazards that may result in contamination [6, 7].

Since food quality and safety are two increasingly interconnected domains, it is of great value to identify which constituents in food make it unfeasible to consume. These components, called contaminants, are increasingly regulated and controlled, because their improper consumption can interfere with consumer health.

In 1963, a harmonized international collection of food standards, guidelines, and codes of practice was created by the Codex Alimentarius Commission, a joint intergovernmental body of the Food Agriculture Organization (FAO) and the World Health Organization (WHO), to protect consumer health and ensure fair food trade practices.

Since contaminants are defined as substances that are not intentionally added to food and may result from various stages such as production, packaging, transport or storage, or environmental factors, the Codex Committee on Contaminants in Food (CCCF) establishes and endorses maximum allowable levels or guideline levels for naturally occurring contaminants and toxins in food and feed. Codex has established 17 maximum levels for these types of substances, including some hazardous metals, mycotoxins produced by certain fungi, and radionuclides [8].

EU legislation, through its Regulations 315/93/EEC [9], 1881/2006 [10], and amendments, imposes procedures for the determination of contaminants and their maximum levels. Thus, in this issue we will cover three main topics related to the intrinsic quality of food, namely heavy metals, polycyclic aromatic hydrocarbons (PAHs), mycotoxins.

There is a wide variety of synthetic and natural organic pollutants found in the environment, contaminating air, water, soils, and therefore, animals and plants, many of them are used for human food. However, within this vast array are the PAHs that present a great structural diversity, possessing two or more benzene rings. These hydrocarbons can be produced by pyrolysis or incomplete combustion of carbon compounds, such as oil and coal [11, 12].

Highly important and problematic is the fact that this group of aromatic organic compounds can be teratogenic, carcinogenic, and mutagenic, can cause serious problems in human health, and can therefore be used as a marker for the occurrence of polycyclic aromatic hydrocarbons in food [13]. Processing of food, such as smoking, heating, and drying processes, and cooking at high temperatures are the major sources of contamination by PAHs because those processes allow combustion products to come into contact with food. High levels of PAH are found in dried fruits, olive pomace oil, teas, smoked fish, grape seed oil, smoked meat products, fresh mollusks, and condiments [12, 14].

Existence of PAH and its relationship with human health and nutrition is an issue that goes back more than half a century. To protect public health, maximum levels are also necessary for foods where environmental pollution may cause high levels of contamination especially in fish and fishery products that contact contaminated water [15]. The detection, identification, monitoring, and regulation that exist today rely on identities such as the Joint FAO/WHO Expert Committee on Food Additives (JECFA), the European Food Safety Authority (EFSA), the Scientific Committee on Food (SCF), the United States Environmental Protection Agency (U.S. EPA), the International Agency for Research on Cancer (IACR), and the International Programme on Chemical Safety (IPCS), that have joined forces to raise alert to this issue [16].

Based on the evaluation of PAHs, in 2002, the European Union through SCF concluded that 15 PAHs, namely benz[a]anthracene, benzo[b]fluoranthene, benzo[j]fluoranthene, benzo[k]fluoranthene, benzo[ghi]perylene, benzo[a]pyrene, chrysene, cyclopenta[cd]pyrene, dibenzo[a,h]anthracene, dibenzo[a,e]pyrene, dibenzo[a,h]pyrene, dibenzo[a,i]pyrene, dibenzo[a,l]pyrene, indeno[1,2,3-cd]pyrene, and 5-methylchrysene showed evidence of mutagenicity, genotoxicity [14]. In 2005, EFSA concluded that benzo[a]pyrene could be used as marker to exposure to, and effect of, genotoxic and carcinogenic PAHs. Later, in 2008, the evaluations showed that 50% of the thousands of samples analyzed contained benzo[a]pyrene, but that 30% of the samples that showed carcinogenic properties contained no benzo[a]pyrene. Based on these and other findings, the CONTAM Panel concluded that the risk characterization should be based upon oral carcinogenicity data of eight PAHs, explicitly benzo[a]pyrene, benz[a]anthracene, benzo[b]fluoranthene, benzo[k]fluoranthene, benzo[ghi]perylene, chrysene, dibenz[a,h]anthracene, and indeno[1,2,3-cd]pyrene (PAH8). These polycyclic aromatic hydrocarbons either individually or in a combination were considered possible indicators of the carcinogenic potency in food. In addition to the effects of the sum of PAH8, the sum of benzo[a]pyrene, chrysene, benz[a]anthracene, and benzo[b]fluoranthene (PAH4), as well as the sum of benzo[a]pyrene and chrysene (PAH2), and the correlation between PAH2, PAH4, and PAH8 were calculated. The CONTAM Panel later concluded that benzo[a]pyrene is not an appropriate indicator for PAH in food and that PAH4 and PAH8 are the most appropriate indicators of PAH in food, with PAH8 not providing much added value compared with PAH4, which are presented in **Table 1** [16, 17].

Polycyclic aromatic hydrocarbons (PAH4)	Other names	Structure
Benzo[a]pyrene	3,4-Benzopyrene 3,4-Bnzpyrene Benzo[*def*]chrysene	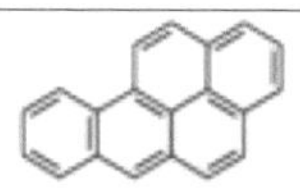
Benz(a)anthracene	1,2-Benzanthracene Tetraphene	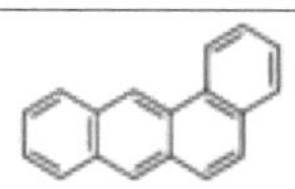
Benzo(b)fluoranthene	2,3-Benzfluoranthene 3,4-Benz[*e*]acephenanthrylene 3,4-Benzfluoranthene 3,4-Benzofluoranthene Benz[*e*]acephenanthrylene Benzo[*e*]fluoranthene	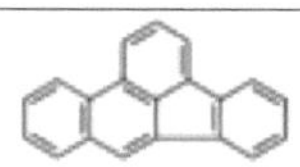
Chrysene	1,2-Benzophenanthrene 1,2-Benzphenanthrene Benzo[a]phenanthrene [4]Phenacene	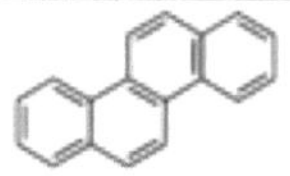

Table 1.
Polycyclic aromatic hydrocarbons (PAH4) and structures.

The foods with maximum levels of PAH4, benzo(a)pyrene, benzo(a)anthracene, benzo(b)fluoranthene and chrysene, above those laid down in EU Regulations 315/93/EEC [9], and 1881/2006 [10] may not be consumed nor used for the edible part of the food. However, recently new data have been collected in order to obtain more useful information on PAHs. An example of this is the new regulated values for powders of food of plant origin used for the preparation of beverages, contained in Regulation 2020/1255 [18], where the maximum thresholds of 10 μg/kg for benzo(a) pyrene and 50 μg/kg for the sum of benzo(a)pyrene, benz(a)anthracene, benzo(b) fluoranthene, and chrysene are established. The same regulation warns of the need to look for new alternative smoking practices to reduce PAH contaminants. This last point is illustrative of the regulators' concern for maintaining food safety, but also shows the concern for food quality, which has great weight at consumer level and also directly in the production and marketing of smoked products and their derivatives.

European Union also establishment, in Commission Regulation (EC) No 1881/2006 [10], the maximum levels for cadmium (Cd), lead, mercury (Hg), inorganic tin (Sn), and arsenic (As), knowing that the exposure of these heavy metals may lead to oxidation stress, which may induce DNA damage, protein modification, lipid peroxidation, and consequently, toxicity in plants and humans [19, 20]. It is important to mention, from a chemical point of view, that arsenic, although being classified as a nonmetal, is included in the group of heavy metals when it comes to environmental parameters. Consequently, from this point on we will roughly call arsenic a heavy metal [21].

For these metallic elements, the European Commission, through Regulation EC No 1881/2006 [10], sets the maximum levels for certain contaminants in foodstuffs, has fixed the tolerable weekly intake (PTWI) of mercury and lead at 1.6 and 25 μg/kg body weight (bw), respectively, Regulation EC No 488/2014 [22] sets the tolerable weekly intake (TWI) at 2.5 μg/kg bw/week for cadmium, and EC Regulation 2015/1006 [23] annexed to the Regulation EC No 1881/2006 [10], estimated maximum dietary exposures BMDL01 between 0.3 and 8 μg/kg bw/day for arsenic.

Chemical contamination is a consumer concern, but microbiological is the greatest one [24]. The presence of mycotoxins in food and feed is an important concern of the authorities concerning food safety and quality, as their presence may have an important impact on the health of consumers both in the short term and in the long term [25]. Due to its toxicity, the Rapid Alert System for Food and Feed (RASFF) in 2017 considered mycotoxins among the top 10 risk categories in terms of contaminants for food and products [26].

Mycotoxins are products resulting from the secondary metabolic by certain filamentous fungi, they are not essential for their growth and reproduction but can cause biochemical, physiological, and pathological changes in many species [27]. Fungi frequently occur in several crops, such as wheat, corn, soybeans, sorghum, and dried fruits, as well as in derived products used in human food and feed; they can accumulate in maturing products already in the field, or during harvesting, in transportation or also in storage [28–30].

Depending on microclimatic conditions, such as moisture content, temperature, pH value, and food matrix composition, fungi can produce more than one mycotoxin, and some mycotoxins are produced by more than one fungal species [31, 32]; once produced they can be modified as a result of interactions between fungi and host or during processing, so when humans or animals are exposed to several mycotoxins simultaneously synergistic effects can be observed [25]. Most mycotoxins are low-molecular-weight compounds (less than 1000 Daltons) [33], highly liposoluble, very stable, and can accumulate over time both during crop growth and post-harvest.

The European Union authorities produce documentation regarding a comprehensive strategy to be implemented by the food production chain in terms of correct pre-harvest management and post-harvest strategies and also on sanitary conditions as well on the technology and operating conditions in live cycle products [25] to prevent and minimize the contents of mycotoxins as a food contaminant [34].

The main fungi producing mycotoxin belonging to the genera *Aspergillus*, *Fusarium*, *Penicillium*, *Claviceps*, *Cladosporium*, *Helminthosporium*, and *Alternaria* [27]. Presently, more than 500 mycotoxins have been identified; however, the ones of most concerns to the agricultural and public health authorities are aflatoxins (AFTs), ochratoxins (OTs), trichothecenes (TCT's), fumonisins (FUMs), zearalenone (ZEN), patulin (PAT), citrinin (CT), and ergot, alkaloids (EAs) [31]. Mycotoxins are very different compounds not only chemically but also toxicologically, so it is practically impossible to systematize them. Nevertheless, from the chemical point of view, the most important ones are classified into cyclopeptides, polycetoacids, terpenes, and nitrogenous metabolites [27].

We can also distinguish between the field toxins, present in the crops, represented mainly by Fusarium deoxynivalelol mycotoxins (DON), zearalenone, fumonisins, and T-2/HT-2 toxins and the storage toxins of which the main ones are aflatoxins (Aflatoxin B1) and ochratoxins (Ochratoxin A).

Human and animals can be exposed to mycotoxins through oral (i.e., dietary consumption) inhalation (dust), and dermal routes, due to their chemical characteristics they are easily absorbed and undergo systemic distribution. In systemic circulation they reach several organs, such as the liver, kidneys, nervous system, and immunological system [33], causing alterations in the immunological response carcinogenicity, teratogenicity, hepatotoxicity, neurotoxicity, nephrotoxicity, reproductive and developmental toxicity, gastrointestinal disorders, among others [32, 35].

Considering that carcinogenic and mutagenic mycotoxin actions are the main health risk in prolonged exposure, Claeys et al. in their systematic review in 2020 [36] classify the main mycotoxins according to International Agency for Research on Cancer (IRCA) criteria into three groups: group 1—The agent is carcinogenic to humans; group 2A—The agent is probably carcinogenic to humans; group 2B—The agent is possibly carcinogenic to humans; group 3—The agent is not classifiable as to its carcinogenic to humans [37]. In **Table 2**, we gather the IARC toxic effects by Claeys et al. with disease-related problem, fungal species, their occurrence, and the limited daily intake, when studied.

The action of mycotoxins as carcinogenic agents is explained by their chemical characteristics, which allow them to easily penetrate both in human and animal cells, reaching the genome, where they can cause mutations in the nucleotide sequence, which can lead to important and permanent alterations in the natural cellular processes of transcription and translation, giving rise to mutations that can exacerbate and deregulate cell growth [32].

According to the above, the study of mycotoxin toxicity goes beyond its carcinogenic and teratogenic effects; its local action in the various systems is of particular importance, aerial topical action at the level of the skin and respiratory system [48–52]. In the digestive system beyond its acute action at the level of vomiting and diarrhea, the effects on microbiota cause changes in the phylum, genus, and microbiota species level of the various animals exposed. The alterations of microbiota have an important consequence on health, as it causes alterations in the composition of short-chain volatile fatty acids and the sphingolipids normally present in the digestive tract; these alterations have been related to the appearance of several chronic diseases in human [35].

Mycotoxins	Toxic effect	Disease-related problem/targeting system	Fungal species	Frequently contaminated products	Maximum tolerable daily intake
Aflatoxins B1, B2, G1, G2 (AFB1, AFB2, AFG1, AFG2) e Aflatoxin M1(AFM1)	IARC Group 1	Liver cancer, immune system	*Aspergillus genus*	Cereals (e.g., sorghum, rice, corn, wheat, barely), oil seed (e.g., cotton, rape, sunflower) nuts (e.g., peanuts, groundnut, pistachio), spices (e.g., turmeric, black and red pepper, ginger), meat, fruit juices, eggs, feed, and foods derived from these products.	<1 ng/g [38]
Ochratoxin A (OTA)	IARC Group 2B	Renal cancer, liver, cardiovascular and immune systems	*Aspergillus* section *Circumdati* *Aspergillus* section *Nigris*, *Penicillium verrucosum*, *Penicillium nordicum*	Soya bean, nuts, red pepper, cereals, green coffee beans, coffee beans Grapes, red pepper, peanuts, cereals dry ham, salami	4 ng/kg bw/day [39]
Fumonisins B1, B2 (FB1, FB2)		Hepatocarcinoma, stimulation and suppression of the immune system, defects in the neural-tube, nephrotoxicity	*Fusarium verticillioides*, *Fusarium proliferatum*, and *Aspergillus nigri*	Peanut, maize, and grape, feed, and foods derived from these products	2 μg/kg bw/day [40]
Sterigmatocystin (STC)		Hepatocellular carcinomas, hemangiosarcomas of the liver and pulmonary adenomas	*Aschersonia*, *Aspergillus*, *Bipolaris*, *Botryotrichum*, *Chaetomium*, *Emericellai*, *Eurotium*, *Farrowia*, *Fusarium*, *Humicola*, *Moelleriella*, *Monocillium*, *Podospora*	Cheese, spices (e.g., turmeric, black, white, red and chilli, pepper, cumin, and marjoram, caraway), cereals (barely, oat, wheat, corn, rice, buckwheat, soybean, sorghum) and derived from cereals (pastas, breakfast cereals)	1.5 μg/kg [41]
Fusarin C		Mutagen and immunosuppressive activities (comparable to aflatoxins B1 and sterigmatocystin) Human esophageal cancer [42]	*Fusarium avenaceum*, *F. culmorum*, *F. fujikuroi*, *F. graminearum*, *Fusarium oxysporum*, *Fusarium poae*, *Fusarium sporotrichioides*, *Fusarium venenatum*, and also by *Metarhizium anisopliae*	Cereals (wheat, oats, barley, and maize), and fruit (banana and pineapple), lentils, tomato, and pea	No available data

Mycotoxins	Toxic effect	Disease-related problem/targeting system	Fungal species	Frequently contaminated products	Maximum tolerable daily intake
Deoxynivalenol (DON)[1]	IARC Group 3	Vomiting, digestive disorders and oxidative damage. Cytotoxicity and genotoxicity.	*Fusarium graminearum*, *F. culmorum* and *F. crookwellense*	Wheat, barley, oats, rye, maize, rice, sorghum and triticale	PMTDI[2], PDI[3] 1 μg/kg bw/day[4] [43]
Zearalenone (ZEN)		Endocrine disruptor (interaction with estrogen-receptors)	*Fusarium graminearum*, *F. culmorum*	Wheat, barley, oats, rye, and maize	PMTDI 0.5 μg/kg bw/day TDI[5] 0.25 μg/kg bw/day (20) [44]
Citrinin (CIT)		Nephrotoxic[6]. Involved in induction of apoptosis though oxidative stress [45]	*Aspergillus*, *Penicillium* and *Monacus*	Mainly in stored grain. Benas, fruit, vegetables herbs and spices	**EU MLs**[7] 2000 μg/kg [46]
Patulin (PAT)		Gastrointestinal ulceration, immunotoxicity and neurotoxicity	*Byssochlamys nivea*, *Penicillium expansum*, *Aspergillus section Clavati*	Fruits especially apples silage	PMTDI 0.4 μg/kg bw/day [44]

A recent study with 3000 Swedish students [47] evaluated the concentrations in urine of various mycotoxins, the data showed a worrying concentration of DON levels.
[2]*PMTDI, provisional maximum tolerable daily intake.*
[3]*PDI, probable daily intake.*
[4]*bw, body weight per day.*
[5]*TDI, tolerable daily intake.*
[6]*The co-occurrence with other mycotoxins, special ochratoxin A, is usually associated with endemic nephropathy.*
[7]*EU MLs, European maximum levels (EFSA).*

Table 2.
Main mycotoxins, toxic effect according to IARC, fungal species, frequently contaminated products, and maximum tolerable daily intake.

It is necessary to process food under standardized and well-controlled conditions and control each food production cycle and storage chain. Preventive measures capable of reducing contamination to a minimum must be implemented. If contamination occurs, methods to reduce or eliminate mycotoxins should be implemented independently of several parameters such as food or feed properties.

The prevalence of mycotoxin in food and feeds calls for the attention of food safety organizations to create awareness on their control and the need to put in place strict regulations to avoid high levels of exposure. Recent studies show that children may be exposed to mycotoxins from the time of breastfeeding resulting from the prevalence of mycotoxins in the mother's diet [32].

2. Conclusion

In fact, food quality is a very broad concept, which, according to Jeantet et al. [53], covers five different components: safety, health, sensory, service, and society, which converge in numerous aspects and criteria. This categorization is much broader than the definition of food quality from the consumer's point of view, which is much narrower, focusing mainly on sensory and health aspects [2]. Thus, when focusing on food quality, it is inevitable to mention food safety, which, in our view, is one of the fundamental bases for consuming quality food. The implementation and application of regulations and standards of good practice in production and processing, the application of sanitary controls, the design of production and processing facilities, and the continuous monitoring of all processes are elements that help reduce the risk of contamination and hygiene that can seriously compromise public health.

Acknowledgements

This research was funded by Fundação para a Ciência e a Tecnologia (FCT, Portugal), through projects UIDP/04567/2020 and UIDB/04567/2020. P.P. gratefully acknowledges the support of the CERENA strategic project FCT-UID/ECI/04028/2019.

Conflict of interest

The authors declare no conflict of interest.

Author details

Marisa Nicolai[1], Paula Pereira[1,2,3] and Lídia Palma[1*]

1 CBIOS—Lusófona University Research Center for Biosciences & Health Technologies, Líbon, Portugal

2 CERENA—Instituto Superior Técnico (IST Center for Natural Resources and Environment), Lisbon University, Líbon, Portugal

3 EPCV—ULHT—Escola de Psicologia e Ciência da Vida, Lusofóna University, Lisbon, Portugal

*Address all correspondence to: lidia.palma@ulusofona.pt

References

[1] Grunert KG, Grunert SC. Measuring subjective meaning structures by the laddering method: Theoretical considerations and methodological problems. International Journal of Research in Marketing. 1995;**12**:209-225

[2] Grunert KG, Frewer LJ, Trijp HC. How consumers perceive food quality. Understanding Consumers of Food Products. 2006:181-199. DOI: 10.1533/9781845692506.2.181

[3] Tothill IE, Stephen S. Methods for environmental monitoring: Biological methods. In: Ahmad R, Cartwright C, Taylor F, editors. Analytical Methods for Environmental Monitoring. Harlow, England: Prentice Hall; 2001. pp. 224-258

[4] Hussain MA. Food contamination: Major challenges of the future foods. Foods. 2016;**5**(2):21. DOI: 10.3390/foods5020021

[5] OECD. Promoting Sustainable Consumption: Good Practices in OECD Countries. Paris, France: Secretary-General the OECD; 2008

[6] FAO. Manual of Food Quality Control: Quality Assurance in the Food Control Microbiological Laboratory. Rome: Food and Agriculture Organization of the United Nations; 1991

[7] FAO and WHO. Food Control System Assessment Tool: Introduction and Glossary. Food Safety and Quality Series No. 7/1. Rome; 2019

[8] FAO/WHO. Codex Alimentarius Food International Standards. 2021. Available from: http://www.fao.org/fao-who-codexalimentarius/en/ [Accessed: 19 February 2021]

[9] Commission Regulation 315/93/EEC of 8 February 1993 on procedures for contaminants in food—EUR-Lex

[10] Commission Regulation EC No 1881/2006 of 19 December 2006 on maximum levels for certain contaminants in food

[11] Singh L, Agarwal T. PAHs in Indian diet: Assessing the cancer risk. Chemosphere. 2018;**202**:366-376. DOI: 10.1016/j.chemosphere.2018.03.100

[12] Guo W, Pan B, Sakkiah S, Yavas G, Ge W, Zou W, et al. Persistent organic pollutants in food: Contamination sources, health effects and detection methods. International Journal of Environmental Research and Public Health. 2019;**16**:4361. DOI: 10.3390/ijerph16224361

[13] Yang J, Lu Z, Liu Z, Wang L, Qiang M. Methylation of imprinted genes in sperm DNA correlated to urinary polycyclic aromatic hydrocarbons (PAHs) exposure levels in reproductive-aged men and the birth outcomes of the offspring. Frontiers in Genetics. 2021;**11**:1-10. DOI: 10.3389/fgene.2020.611276

[14] Bansal V, Kumar P, Kwon EE, Kim K-H. Review of the quantification techniques for polycyclic aromatic hydrocarbons (PAHs) in food products. Critical Reviews in Food Science and Nutrition. 2017;**57**(15):3297-3312. DOI: 10.1080/10408398.2015.1116970

[15] Sun Y, Wu S, Gong G. Trends of research on polycyclic aromatic hydrocarbons in food: A 20-year perspective from 1997 to 2017. Trends in Food Science & Technology. 2019;**83**: 86-98

[16] Zelinkova Z, Wenzl T. The occurrence of 16 EPA PAHs in food—A review. Polycyclic Aromatic Compounds. 2015;**35**:248-284. DOI: 10.1080/10406638.2014.918550

[17] European Food Safety Authority (EFSA). Annual Report. 2008. Available from: http://www.efsa.europa.eu/en/corporate/pub/ar08 [Accessed: 27 February 2021]

[18] Commission Regulation EC No 20/1255 of 07 September 2020 on amending Regulation (EC) No 1881/2006 regards maximum levels of polycyclic aromatic hydrocarbons (PAHs) in traditionally smoked meat and smoked meat products and traditionally smoked fish and smoked fishery products and establishing a maximum level of PAHs in powders of food of plant origin used for the preparation of beverages (text with EEA relevance)

[19] Shahid M, Pourrut B, Dumat C, Nadeem M, Aslam M, Pinelli E. Heavy-metal-induced reactive oxygen species: Phytotoxicity and physicochemical changes in plants. Reviews of Environmental Contamination and Toxicology. 2014;**232**:1-44. DOI: 10.1007/978-3-319-06746-9_1

[20] Wu X, Cobbina SJ, Mao G, et al. A review of toxicity and mechanisms of individual and mixtures of heavy metals in the environment. Environmental Science and Pollution Research. 2016;**23**:8244-8259. DOI: 10.1007/s11356-016-6333-x

[21] Pereira P, Palma C, Ferreira-Pêgo C, Amaral O, Amaral A, Rijo P, et al. Grape pomace: A safe potential ingredient for the human diet. Food. 2020;**9**(12):1772. DOI: 10.3390/foods9121772

[22] Commission Regulation EC No 488/2014 of 12 May 2014 on amending Regulation (EC) No 1881/2006 as regards maximum levels of cadmium in foodstuffs

[23] Commission Regulation EC 2015/1006 of 25 June 2015 on amending Regulation (EC) No 1881/2006 as regards maximum levels of inorganic arsenic in foodstuffs

[24] Bruhn CM. Consumer perceptions and concerns about food contaminants. In: Jackson LS, Knize MG, Morgan JN, editors. Impact of Processing on Food Safety (Advances in Experimental Medicine and Biology). Vol. 459. Boston, MA: Springer; 1999. DOI: 10.1007/978-1-4615-4853-9_1

[25] Battilani P, Palumbo R, Giorni P, Dall'Asta C, Dellafiora L, Gkrillas A, et al. Mycotoxin mixtures in food and feed: Holistic, innovative, flexible risk assessment modelling approach. EFSA Supporting Publications. 2020;**17**(1):1757E

[26] Guillermina F, Ruiz M. Editorial: Mechanism of mycotoxins. Food and Chemical Toxicology. 2019;**123**:520-521. DOI: 10.1016/j.fct.2018.11.044

[27] Pleadin J, Frece J, Markov K. Mycotoxins in food and feed. Advances in Food and Nutrition Research. 2019;**89**:297-345. DOI: 10.1016/bs.afnr.2019.02.007

[28] Bilandžić N, Božić DD, Dokić M, Sedak M, Kolanović BS, Varenina I, et al. Seasonal effect on aflatoxin M1 contamination in raw and UHT milk from Croatia. Food Control. 2014;**40**(1):260-264

[29] Chiotta ML, Fumero MV, Cendoya E, Palazzini JM, Alaniz-Zanon MS, Ramirez ML, et al. Toxigenic fungal species and natural occurrence of mycotoxins in crops harvested

in Argentina. Revista Argentina de Microbiología. 2020;**52**(4):339-347

[30] Fernanda C, Cebin Coppa S, Khaneghah AM, Alvito P, Assunção R, Martins C, et al. The occurrence of mycotoxins in breast milk, fruit products and cereal-based infant formula: A review. Trends in Food Science and Technology. 2019;**92**:81-93. DOI: 10.1016/j.tifs.2019.08.014

[31] Haque MA, Wang Y, Shen Z, Li X, Saleemi MK, He C. Mycotoxin contamination and control strategy in human, domestic animal and poultry: A review. Microbial Pathogenesis. 2020;**142**:104095. DOI: 10.1016/j.micpath.2020.104095

[32] Adegbeye MJ, Reddy PRK, Chilaka CA, Balogun OB, Elghandour MMMY, Rivas-Caceres RR, et al. Mycotoxin toxicity and residue in animal products: Prevalence, consumer exposure and reduction strategies—A review. Toxicon. 2020;**177**:96-108. DOI: 10.1016/j.toxicon.2020.01.007

[33] Alshannaq AYJ-H. Occurrence, toxicity, and analysis of major mycotoxins in food. International Journal of Environmental Research and Public Health. 2017;**14**(623):1-20

[34] EFSA Funds Project Evaluating Mycotoxin Co-occurrence Risk Analysis Tools [Internet]. Available from: https://www.feednavigator.com/Article/2017/02/24/EFSA-funds-project-evaluating-mycotoxin-co-occurrence-risk-analysis-tools [Cited: 2 February 2021]

[35] Guerre P. Mycotoxin and gut microbiota interactions. Toxins (Basel). 2020;**12**(12):1-33

[36] Claeys L, Romano C, De Ruyck K, et al. Mycotoxin exposure and human cancer risk: A systematic review of epidemiological studies. Comprehensive Reviews in Food Science and Food Safety. 2020;**19**(4):1449-1464

[37] Agents Classified by the IARC Monographs, Volumes 1-128—IARC Monographs on the Identification of Carcinogenic Hazards to Humans [Internet]. Available from: https://monographs.iarc.who.int/agents-classified-by-the-iarc/ [Cited: 28 February 2021]

[38] Noreddine B. Aflatoxins: Producing-molds, structure, health issues and incidence in Southeast Asian and Sub-Saharan African countries. International Journal of Environmental Research and Public Health. 2020;**17**(1215):1-40

[39] Malir F, Ostry V, Pfohl-Leszkowicz A, Malir J, Toman J. Ochratoxin A: 50 years of research. Toxins (Basel). 2016;**8**(7):12-15

[40] Kamle M, Mahato DK, Devi S, Lee KE, Kang SG, Kumar P. Fumonisins: Impact on agriculture, food, and human health and their management strategies. Toxins (Basel). 2019;**11**(6):1-23

[41] Díaz Nieto CH, Granero AM, Zon MA, Fernández H. Sterigmatocystin: A mycotoxin to be seriously considered. Food and Chemical Toxicology. 2018;**118**:460-470

[42] Perincherry L, Lalak-Kánczugowska J, Stepién L. Fusarium-produced mycotoxins in plant-pathogen interactions. Toxins (Basel). 2019;**11**(664):1-22

[43] Chen L, Yu M, Wu Q, Peng Z, Wang D, Kuča K, et al. Gender and geographical variability in the exposure pattern and metabolism of deoxynivalenol in humans: A review. Journal of Applied Toxicology. 2017;**37**(1):60-70

[44] Robert H, Payros D, Pinton P, Théodorou V, Mercier-Bonin M, Oswald IP. Impact of mycotoxins on the intestine: Are mucus and microbiota new targets? Journal of Toxicology and Environmental Health, Part B: Critical Reviews. 2017;**20**(5):249-275. DOI: 10.1080/10937404.2017.1326071

[45] Čulig B, Bevardi M, Bošnir J, Serdar S, Lasić D, Racz A, et al. Presence of citrinin in grains and its possible health effects. African Journal of Traditional, Complementary, and Alternative Medicines. 2017;**14**(3): 22-30

[46] Ali N. Co-occurrence of citrinin and ochratoxin A in rice in Asia and its implications for human health. Journal of the Science of Food and Agriculture. 2018;**98**(6):2055-2059

[47] Warensjö Lemming E, Montano Montes A, Schmidt J, Cramer B, Humpf HU, Moraeus L, et al. Mycotoxins in blood and urine of Swedish adolescents—Possible associations to food intake and other background characteristics. Mycotoxin Research. 2020;**36**(2):193-206

[48] Cai GH, Hashim JH, Hashim Z, Ali F, Bloom E, Larsson L, et al. Fungal DNA, allergens, mycotoxins and associations with asthmatic symptoms among pupils in schools from Johor Bahru, Malaysia. Pediatric Allergy and Immunology. 2011;**22**(3):290-297

[49] Norbäck D, Hashim JH, Cai GH, Hashim Z, Ali F, Bloom E, et al. Rhinitis, ocular, throat and dermal symptoms, headache and tiredness among students in schools from Johor Bahru, Malaysia: Associations with fungal DNA and mycotoxins in classroom dust. Science of The Total Environment. 2016:545-546, 95-103

[50] Capcarova M, Zbynovska K, Kalafova A, Bulla J, Bielik P. Environment contamination by mycotoxins and their occurrence in food and feed: Physiological aspects and economical approach. Journal of Environmental Science and Health - Part B Pesticides, Food Contaminants, and Agricultural Wastes. 2016;**51**(4):236-244

[51] Kadawathagedara M, De Lauzon-Guillain B, Botton J. Environmental contaminants and child's growth. Journal of Developmental Origins of Health and Disease. 2018;**9**(6):632-641

[52] Hurraß J, Heinzow B, Aurbach U, Bergmann KC, Bufe A, Buzina W, et al. Medical diagnostics for indoor mold exposure. International Journal of Hygiene and Environmental Health. 2017;**220**(2):305-328

[53] Jeantet R, Croquennec T, Schuck P, Brulé G. Handbook of Food Science and Technology 1: Food Alteration and Food Quality. London, United Kingdom: Wiley-ISTE; 2016

Chapter 3

Mycotoxins ... Silent Death

Azhar A. Alhaddad

Abstract

There are many types of fungi that produce secondary metabolites called mycotoxins. These compounds are very dangerous to humans and animals, as exposure to them causes acute or chronic toxicity. Temperature, humidity and pH are important environmental factors in the production of mycotoxins. There are about 500 types of mycotoxins that are found in many agricultural products such as peanut, cereals, wines, fruit juice, dried fruits, feed, and other foodstuffs. Among the most important genera of fungi that produce mycotoxins are *Aspergillus*, *Penicillium*, *Altenaria*, *Fusarium*, and others. Some of them infect plants in the field and produce mycotoxin, while others infect agricultural crops, foodstuffs, and feed in the store and produce mycotoxin during storage conditions. Mycotoxins are divided into various groups according to the degree of their impact and danger, into highly toxic, low toxic, carcinogenic, and mutagenic. This is depends on the chemical composition of the different types of mycotoxins, which are an open hydrocarbon chain with low molecular weights ranging between 100 and 697 Da. The biological effects of mycotoxins include damage to living tissues, suppression of immunity, and neurological disorders. Aflatoxins are one of the most dangerous mycotoxins as they are the main cause of hepatocellular carcinoma and the fifth most common carcinogen in the world.

Keywords: mycotoxins, characteristics, effects on health

1. Introduction

Mycotoxins are secondary metabolites produced by some fungi that are genetically capable of producing toxins when appropriate environmental and nutritional conditions exist for their production [1]. They are produced by fungi or filamentous molds belonging to the class Ascomycota, have low molecular weights, and are of great importance to human and animal health because they cause acute or chronic toxicity [2]. Directly or indirectly, living vertebrate organisms such as humans and animals are affected when exposed to very low concentrations of mycotoxins [3]. Many mycotoxins play a major role against plant defenses, some of which enable the fungi to compete with the environment in nature. There are hundreds of mycotoxins, some of which are used as the antibiotics we are familiar with, such as penicillin, and others are very dangerous such as aflatoxin, one of the most potent substances known to cause cancer. It is followed by diacetoxyserpineol in a small percentage [4]. The origin of the word mycotoxins is derived from the Greek mykes, meaning fungi, and toxicum, the Latin for poison [5]. Mycotoxins are considered one of the health and economic problems in the world, as they constitute 25% of the problems of field crops. These toxins are found in many agricultural crops, foodstuffs, and feed, which may appear fit for consumption, but they contain many fungi and their secondary metabolites, according to FAO and WHO [6]. Mycotoxins are classified according to the fungi that produce them, their structural properties, and their toxic effects. There are about 400 types of them that vary in their toxicity [7]. Mycotoxins have been associated with diseases throughout history. In 1940s and 1950s of the last century, episodes appeared for humans in Russia and Japan, as intoxication by *Stachybotrys* appeared in the United States of America, and facial eczema appeared in sheep in New Zealand in 1961, In England, many animals died after eating feed polluted, all these events led to the discovery of mycotoxins [8]. Aflatoxins are one of the most important mycotoxins secreted by several genera of fungi such as *Aspergillus*, *Penicillium*, *Fusarium*, in addition to *Alternaria,* as these grow in the temperature range between 10 and 40°C, and these conditions may change according to the type of fungus [7] produced by many types of fungi, or one type of fungi can produce multiple types of mycotoxins, and among the most important and common toxins are Afatoxins of all kinds such as AFB1, AFB2, AFG1, AFG2, and Ochratoxin A (OTA) produced by *Aspergillus* and *Penicillium*, followed by fumonisin FBs such as fumonisinB1 (FB1), fumonisin B2 (FB2), are predominant zearalenone (ZEA) and trichothecenes, the most famous of which are deoxynivalenol (DON) and HT-2 and T-2 toxins. These fungi are associated with the climate and different stages of field crops in addition to geographical areas. Among the common fungi that infect crops in the field and during storage are *Fusarium*, *Alternaria*, *Penicillium*, and *Aspergillus* [9]. Consequently, mycotoxins OTA and AFs are produced in the pre- and postharvest periods, while FBs and DON are mainly produced in the preharvest period, in any type of agricultural crops and their harvesting stages, the presence of mycotoxins can be observed depending on the stage of production of mycotoxins by the fungi, the production of toxins can be reduced. The fungal infection is by following good agricultural practices and methods of controlling them, producing resistant cultivars, and using chemical protection, Despite the different factors suitable for the growth of different types of fungi and their production of mycotoxins, mycotoxins were found in many food and feed samples in the world, as they caused many problems. It travels through the food chain and is mainly found in grain samples and in dairy products, coffee, spices, vegetable oils, dried fruits, nuts, wine, as well as fruit juices [10, 11].

2. The fungi are responsible for producing most of the mycotoxins

If we look at the spread of fungi in foods around the world, which may be able to produce mycotoxins, these fungi contaminated with field crops are divided into two groups, which are:

1. **Field fungi** such as *Cladosporium spp.*, *Fusarium spp.* and *Alternaria spp.*, which infect the whole plant and reach seeds during plant growth and development.

2. **Storage fungi** such as *Aspergillus ssp.* and *Penicillium spp.*, which grow and reproduce during the storage phase [12].

DOI: http://dx.doi.org/10.5772/intechopen.104382

There are four types of toxic fungi that can be distinguished into:

1. Plant pathogens such as *Fusarium graminearum* and *Alternaria alternate.*

2. Fungi grow and produce mycotoxins on large and vulnerable plants such as *Aspergillus flavus* and *Fusarium moniliforme.*

3. Fungi infest the plant and increase its susceptibility to postharvest pollution such as *A. flavus.*

4. Fungi found in the soil, on decaying plants and the remains of field crops, which grow and multiply later during the storage phase, such as *P. verrucosum* and *A. ochraceus* [13].

3. Genus *Aspergillus*

Aspergillus spp. It is one of the plant pathogens that infect crops in the soil from time to time and produces aflatoxin, and the risk of producing aflatoxin increases during wrong agricultural practices, as it was found that *A. flavus* and *A. parasiticus* infect crops before harvest [2]. These species are considered the most important producers of aflatoxins, while Ochratoxins A are produced by *A. ochraceus*, *A. carbonarius*, and *A. niger.* The main species, such as *A. flavus* and *A. parasiticus*, are observed to produce aflatoxins with 10 other types of *Aspergillus* that are rarely found in food. It was found that there is a new species affecting peanuts, *A. minisclerotigenes*, similar to some strains of *A. flavus*, sometimes producing small sclerotia and similar to *A. parasiticus* by producing both Aflatoxins B and G. There is a species associated with insects, but it was found recently on the Brazilian nuts, which is *A. nomius*, as it is similar to *A. flavus* in terms of its production of types B and G and forms bullet-shaped sclerotia [14]. The minimum growth temperature for *A. flavus* ranges between 10 and 12°C and the maximum from 43 to 48°C. The optimum temperature is about 33°C [15]. The minimum aqueous activity (aw) that allows fungus growth is 0.82 at 25°C, 0.81 at 30°C, and 0.80 at 37°C [16]. Optimal growth of the fungus occurs in the pH range of 3.4–10, As for *A. parasiticus*, it grows in the same physical factors as *A. flavus* that were mentioned previously except that the minimum temperature is 42°C [17].

4. Genus *Penicillium*

Penicillium is one of the most common fungi as it is found in different environments such as different field crops, soil, and air. It is also found in food and has a great economic impact on human life. The main role of *Penicillium* is to spoil organic matter. *Penicillium* species are pre- and postharvest pathogens. With rotting of many foodstuffs, this genus is of great importance in many and varied fields such as food spoilage, biotechnology, plant pathology, and medicine [18, 19]. Currently, there are 438 accepted species, most of which are classified as pre- and postharvest pathogens and lead to significant losses in field crops [20]. *Penicillium spp.* are mesophilic fungi, growing between 5 and 37°C (optimal growth of 20–30°C) and at pH 3–4.5, maximum growth was obtained in vitro at 23°C and pH 3–4.5. *Penicillium* genus includes many species, including *Penicillium atramentosum*, *Penicillium digitatum*, *Penicillium expansum*, *Penicillium notatum*, *Penicillium roquefortii*, *Penicillium oxalicum*, *Penicillium glaucum*, and others (https://www.inspq.qc.ca/en/moulds/fact-sheets/*penicillium-spp*). Some species of *Penicillium* produce different types of mycotoxins that cause acute or chronic toxicity to humans, such as Indole-diterpenes, Penitrems (PNT) A, C, F, Patulin (PTA), Citrinin (CTN), Cyclopiazonic acid (CPA), Ochratoxin A (OTA), Penicillic acid (PA), and other mycotoxins [21]. *Penicillium* can produce a variety of secondary metabolites and many antibacterial and antifungal compounds, immune suppressants, as well as cholesterol-lowering agents, the most famous example being penicillin, which was the first historically known antifungal antibiotic [22].

5. Genus *Fusarium*

Fusarium is among the most economically important genera of fungi in the world and is one of the most studied [23]. Most of the species of *Fusarium* live in the soil, *Fusarium conidia* can spread by rain spray or irrigation, but when dry it can spread by air, and this makes it perfectly suitable for long-distance atmospheric dispersal, and this contributes to its distribution all over the world [24]. The optimum temperature range for growth and reproduction of some species *of Fusarium* such as *F. oxysporum* was 24–28°C. The minimum growth is obtained at 45°C and 10°C. Also, the optimum pH for fungal growth was obtained at a pH of 5.5 [25]. *Fusarium spp*. has a very important role for humankind as plant pathogens, and this leads to its real role in creating toxicological risks to humans and our domestic animal species, A wide range of plant diseases are associated with *Fusarium*; most plant-pathogenic *Fusarium spp*. are grouped into four species complexes as defined by RNA polymerase II subunit gene sequence phylogeny such as *Fusarium fujikuroi*, *Fusarium graminearum*, *Fusarium oxysporum*, and *Fusarium solani* [26]. There are many hundreds of compounds (secondary metabolites) secreted by *Fusarium spp.* Described as toxic or potentially toxic, such as Trichothecenes and Fumonisins, these can contaminate agricultural products and make them unsuitable for food or feed. Trichothecenes can also act as virulence factors in plant diseases [27, 28]. There are other mycotoxins produced by some Fusarium spp. It is commonly found in corn and is called Zearalenone (Zea), Its name is a collection of letters from different origins (Zea) comes from *Gibberella zeae*, which is the name of a producing organism that was the first to be studied [29]. There are other species of *Fusarium* producing other types of mycotoxins such as *F. crookwellense* and *F. sambucinum* produce fusaric acid [30]. Moniliformin is produced from *F. moniliforme*, *F. acuminatum*, *F. culmorum*, *F. equiseti*, and *F. sporotrichioides* [31].

6. Characteristics of mycotoxins

Mycotoxins are toxic chemical compounds produced by molds, and molds cannot be used as building blocks for the body of fungi, but they are produced for other reasons that are not clearly understood so far. Fungi compete for their ecological position in nature. There are hundreds of mycotoxins, some of which are used as antibiotics, such as penicillin, others are very dangerous such as aflatoxin, which is one of the most potent carcinogens known, and others, such as diacetoxiscerinol, are much less a favor [32]. Mycotoxins are distinguished toxic chemical compounds produced by fungi. Most mycotoxins are Aromatic hydrocarbon seldom Aliphatic hydrocarbon. With low molecular weights ranging between 100 and 697 Da [33], so they do not stimulate the immune system creating antibodies. Due to the different chemical composition, some may exhibit different biological effects. It causes tissue damage, immunosuppression, and nervous disorders [34]. It dissolves well in organic solvents and is resistant to freezing and high temperatures as boiling point and pasteurization [35]. They resist decomposition during the digestive processes that they occur in the human gastrointestinal system and animal [36]. Mycotoxins differ from each other in the degree of their toxicity. Depending on its chemical composition and molecular construction, as it enters the human body in several ways For example, orally through consuming it with food or inhalation of fungi produced. For toxins through the respiratory system or from by direct contact with fungi producing mycotoxins [37].

7. Some mycotoxins commonly found in food and feed

Mycotoxins exist in agricultural commodities such as peanuts, grapes, wines, grains, nuts, dried fruit, coffee, cocoa, spices, oil seeds, fruits, fruit juices, beer, and other foodstuffs and feed crops, both in the field and during transportation [38–40]. At any stage of the food production process (before harvesting, harvesting, drying, and storage), fungal production of mycotoxins can occur and can expose consumers to the risk of contamination directly through food consumption or indirectly through feed [41]. In general, under prolonged storage conditions and at extreme temperatures along with extreme humidity, all crops including cereals can be subjected to mold growth and mycotoxin contamination [42]. In fact, the occurrence of mycotoxins in foods and derivatives is not only a problem in countries, mycotoxins affect agribusiness in many countries, influencing or even impeding exportation, reducing livestock and crop farming production, and affecting human and animal health [43]. Most of the mycotoxins remain chemically and thermally stable, and this has been observed through various techniques in food processing such as cooking, boiling, baking, frying, and pasteurization, The presence of mycotoxins in animal products such as meat, eggs, and milk is the result of contaminated feed, and this leads to the contamination of the human plate [38]. The agricultural industry has to deal with the presence of mycotoxins in food, as it is of global importance and a major threat [44]. Huge agricultural and industrial losses in billions of dollars occur annually because 25% of the world's harvested crops are contaminated by mycotoxins [45]. The report stressed the WHO and IJRC that there is a need for a coordinated international response to the problem of mycotoxins and contamination of food and neglect of its health effect for a long time It causes human liver cancer, death, and stunting in young children, There are approximately 500 million poor people in sub-Saharan Africa, Latin America, and Asia daily exposed to natural toxins, aflatoxins and fumonisins, by following a diet based mainly on peanuts, corn, and other grains, and this exposure to toxins occurs throughout life as toxin levels far exceed internationally accepted standards, and this is in stark contrast to the situation in developed countries [46].

8. Aflatoxin

Aflatoxins are a type of mycotoxin produced by *Aspergillus* species of fungi, such as *A. flavus* and *A. parasiticus*, The most potent carcinogens found in nature, aflatoxins are toxic not only to humans, but also to livestock, pets, and wildlife [47]. Dietary exposure to aflatoxins is one of the major causes of hepatocellular carcinoma, the fifth most common cancer in humans worldwide [48]. The term aflatoxin was created based on the name of its main agent producer *A. flavus*. The main known aflatoxins are called B1, B2, G1, and G2, based on their fluorescence under ultraviolet light and their mobility during thin layer chromatography (TLC). They are mainly produced by *A. flavus* and *A. parasiticus*. However, more recently, the species *A. nomius*, *A. bombycis*, and *A. tamarii* have also been shown to be aflatoxigenic [49]. More than 20 types of aflatoxins (AFs) and their derivatives occur in nature, but mainly four, B1, B2, G1, and G2, are proved to be dangerous for humans and livestock [50]. Aflatoxins are immunotoxic, carcinogen, and mutagen. The presence of the lactone and devoran ring is mainly due to the effects [51]. AFB1 is considered one of the most studied carcinogens, AFM1 is a 4-hydroxy derivative of AFB1, which is formed in the liver and secreted by the mammary glands in humans and lactating animals when fed a contaminated diet [52]. The chemical formula of the aflatoxin is C17H12O6, colorless to pale yellow crystals. Aflatoxins are soluble in organic solvents such as chloroform and methanol and slightly soluble in water, but insoluble in nonpolar solutions such as phenyl, cyclohexyl, ethyl, octyl, and octadecyl [53, 54] Aflatoxins (AFTs) are derivatives of difuranocoumarin, with a bifuran group attached to one side of the coumarin nucleus while a pentanone ring bound to the other side for AFTs and AFTs-B or six lacton rings attached to the AFTs-G series **Figure 1** [55, 56].

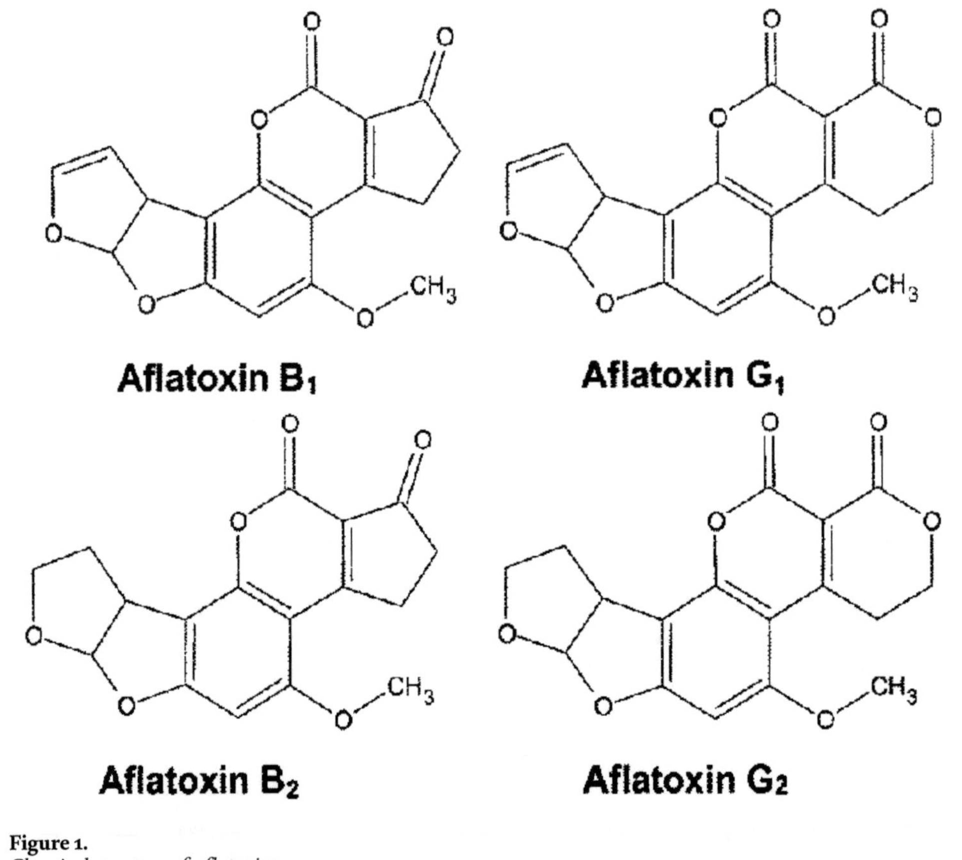

Figure 1.
Chemical structure of aflatoxins.

9. Trichothecenes

Fusarium toxins are produced by over 50 species of *Fusarium* and have a history of infecting the grain of developing cereals such as wheat and maize [57]. They include a range of mycotoxins, such as trichothecenes, which are most strongly associated with chronic and fatal toxic effects in animals and humans, the genera producing trichothecenes include *Fusarium*, *Myrothecium*, *Spicellum*, *Stachybotrys*, and *Cephalosporium*, *Trichoderma,* and *Trichostium*. Trichothecene (TCT) mycotoxin is agriculturally more important worldwide due to the potential health hazards they pose [58, 59]. It produces more than 20 metabolites mainly after the metabolism of trichothecene,

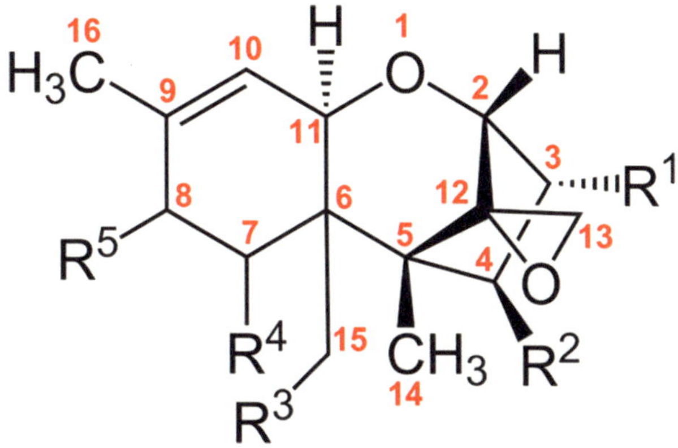

Figure 2.
Chemical structure of trichothecenes.

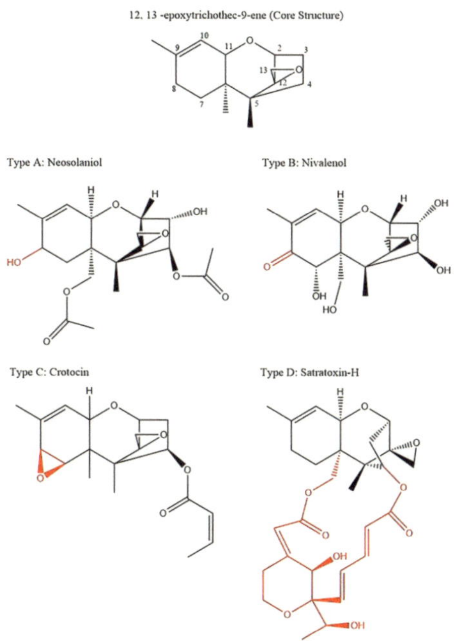

Figure 3.
Chemical structure of trichothecenes types A, B, C, D.

and this happens when ingested to get rid of it, and hydroxy trichothecene-2 is the main metabolite, this family is divided into four groups according to its composition, namely A, B, C, and D [60, 61]). Trichothecenes are groups of chemicals such as T-2 toxin (T-2), HT-2 toxin (HT-2), neosolaniol (NEO), diacetoxyscirpenol (DAS), monoacetoxyscirpenol (MAS), verrucarol (VER), scirpentriol (SCP), and their derivatives are reported as representative type A trichothecenes [62]. Types C and D of trichothecenes are chemical compounds of different structures. It is not produced by *Fusarium* species. Therefore, type A and type B are some of the most common types of trichothecenes found in nature and highly toxic, The most toxic group is type A (T-2 and HT-2) compared with type B DON, NIV, and FUS-X [63, 64]. Trichothcinate is a low-molecular-weight (MW 250–550) mycotoxin, nonvolatile, and slightly soluble in water, but highly soluble in acetone, ethyl acetate, chloroform, dimethyl sulfoxide (DMSO), ethanol, methanol, and propylene glycol Pure trichothcinates have a low vapor pressure but evaporate when heated in organic solvents (**Figures 2** and **3**) [65].

10. Patulin

Patulin (PAT) is produced by many different molds, predominantly by *Penicillium spp*., but, occasionally, by some *Byssochlamys* and *Aspergillus spp*. including *A. giganteus*, *A. longivesica*, and *A. clavatus* [66–68]. It is a low-molecular-weight mycotoxin. Compounds with low volatility, which are secondary metabolites found in crops, in the field or after harvest, are capable of causing disease and death to humans and animals by eating contaminated food products [67]. The contamination of patulin in fruits, vegetables, and fruit-derived products, especially in apple and derived products, is very common worldwide and occasionally in other fruits such as pears, oranges, grapes, and their products [69]. If rotten fruits, especially apples, are not removed during fruit juice processing, patulin is transferred to juices [70]. Patulin is a polycystic metabolite, like many other major mycotoxins, such as aflatoxins, fumonisins, and ochratoxins, but this latter toxin is a polycetoxin/amino acid hybrid compound, Structurally, PAT is a heterocyclic lactone (4-hidroxi-4H-furo [3,2-c] piran-2(6H)-ona) (**Figure 4**) [71].

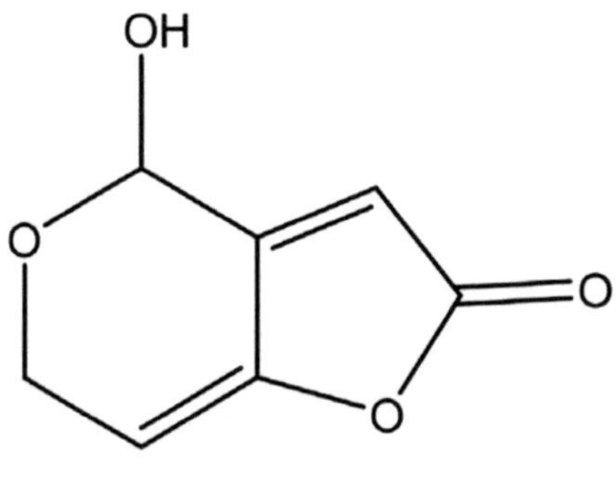

$C_7H_6O_4$ - molecular weight = 154.12 g/mol

Figure 4.
Chemical structure of patulin.

11. Mycotoxins and public health

There are approximately 500 mycotoxins, most of which have been discovered since the 1960s, it has been generally classified into groups based on structural similarities and its major toxic effects [56]. Mycotoxins are classified into polycetoacids, cyclopeptides, terpenes, and nitrogenous metabolites, depending on their biological origin and structure. From a health point of view, the important mycotoxins in food and feed include: aflatoxins, ochratoxin, trichothecenes, fumonisins, ZEN, and patulin. Aaflatoxins, fumonisins, and ergot alkaloids are associated with acute mycotoxicoses in both humans and livestock [72]. Mycotoxins can travel through the food chains of humans and animals through direct or indirect contamination, The indirect contamination of food and animal feed occurs when any component has been previously contaminated with toxic fungi, and mycotoxins remain in the final product despite the elimination of the fungi during processing, on the other hand, direct contamination occurs when the product, food, or feed is infected with a fungus toxic with the subsequent formation of mycotoxins. It is known that most food and feed products can allow toxin-causing fungi to grow and develop during production, processing, transport, and storage [7]. The term mycotoxicosis is given to the toxic effect of mycotoxins on human and animal health. Mostly exposure to mycotoxins is through ingestion but can also occur through inhalation and skin. The extent of harmful effects of mycotoxins on human and animal health depends mainly on exposure (dose and period). The physiological and nutritional status, the type of toxins, as well as the potential synergistic effects of other chemical substances to which humans or animals are exposed [73]. Aflatoxins are the best known among all mycotoxins, because of their serious impact on human and animal health, aflatoxin.

B1 is a carcinogenic substance (according to the classification by the IARC in 1987, while AFM1 is a potentially carcinogenic substance with a toxicity range of B1, G1, B2, and G2 [74, 75]. In addition to being a carcinogen, aflatoxin is mutagenic (DNA destruction), have teratogenic effects, and immunosuppressive effects. Symptoms of acute aflatoxicosis in humans include vomiting, abdominal pain, jaundice, pulmonary edema, coma, convulsions, and death while chronic aflatoxicosis occurs via cancer, immune system inhibition, and liver damage [76, 77]. Aflatoxicosis is the consumption of foods or feed contaminated with high levels of aflatoxins, which leads to acute Aflatoxicosis, while regular intake at low levels (ppb) is responsible for stunting and weight loss in children and in some cases led to the development of hepatocellular carcinoma. Aflatoxins have also been linked with kwashiorkor, a protein-energy malnutrition disease [78]. Those who are most exposed to Aflatoxicosis illness are residents of developing countries, because the security blankets on crops before and after harvest is not as strict as in other countries.

The same is happening with dairy products, as developing countries do not accept or assume amenities like developed countries, and it is estimated that there are more than 5 billion people in developing countries around the world at risk of chronic exposure to aflatoxins through contaminated foods [79]. The effects of aflatoxins are similar in all animals; however, susceptibility to infection varies by gender, age, and individual variation. Symptoms of acute poisoning consist of depression, loss of appetite, weight loss, disease, gastrointestinal bleeding, and pulmonary edema

Liver damage. Signs of acute liver injury are thrombosis and capillary enlargement feeling, bleeding, and prolonged clotting. Pigments of blood may appear in urine and mucous membranes are rhythmic. Symptoms of prolonged exposure to moderate to aflatoxins may be reflected in a decline in feed consumption and production (growth and production of eggs and milk) [80]. The US Food and Drug Administration (FDA) has recommended acceptable levels of aflatoxins in foods and feeds in order to protect human and animal health from the toxicity of high doses of aflatoxins, The permissible levels range from 20 to 300 ppm, depending on the product and host (children, adults, animals) **Table 1** [81]. Trichothecenes are toxic to humans, other mammals, birds, fish, plants, and plants Eukaryotic cells in general, TCT is dangerously toxic due to its added ability to be locally absorbed. Its metabolites affect the gastrointestinal tract, kidneys, liver, skin, cellular immune system, and blood. The most sensitive end points are in neuroimmune effects, hematological and reproductive diseases, and there is variation in the sensitivity of some animals. This type of poison ranges from dairy cows to pigs [82]. The mechanism of action mainly consists of the inhibition of protein synthesis and oxidative damage to cells followed by the disruption of nucleic acid synthesis and ensuing apoptosis [59]). Trichothecenes have a spectrum of adverse effects including emesis, anorexia, growth retardation, neuroendocrine changes, immunotoxicity, and a reduction in food consumption in various animal species (mink, mice, and pigs) [83]. TCT is easily absorbed in the membranes of the gastrointestinal tract and is rapidly distributed to various organs and tissues of the

Aflatoxin		
Commodity	**Action level (ppb)**	**Reference**
Animal feeds		
Brazil nuts	20	CPG 570.200
Foods	20	CPG 555.400
Milk	0.5 (aflatoxin M1)	CPG 527.400
Peanuts and peanut products	20	CPG 570.375
Pistachio nuts	20	CPG 570.500
Corn, peanut products, and other animal feeds and feed ingredients but excluding cottonseed meal, intended for immature animals	20	CPG 683.100
Corn, peanut products, cottonseed meal, and other animal feed ingredients intended for dairy animals, for animal species or uses not specified above, or when the intended use is not known	20	CPG 683.100
Corn and peanut products intended for breeding beef cattle, breeding swine, or mature poultry	100	CPG 683.100
Corn and peanut products intended for finishing swine of 100 pounds or greater	200	CPG 683.100
Corn and peanut products intended for finishing (i.e., feedlot) beef cattle	300	CPG 683.100
Cottonseed meal intended for beef, cattle, swine, or poultry (regardless of age or breeding status	300	CPG 683.100

Table 1.
FDA action levels for aflatoxins present in animal feeds and food.

body due to its low molecular weight and amphipathic nature. The toxic activity of trichothecenes is due to the fact that they all contain epoxide at the C12,13 position [84]. Modulation of emesis and anorexia occur as a result of the direct action of trichothecenes in the brain or the indirect action in the gastrointestinal tract. The direct action of trichothecenes is in specific areas of the brain such as nucleate tractus solitarius in the brainstem and the arcuate nuclei in the hypothalamus. Activation of these areas in the brain leads to the activation of specific neuronal populations containing anorexigenic factors [85]. Since trichothecenes induce emesis and growth retardation, mycotoxin contamination is becoming a major issue for child and young animal health [86]. The trichothecene mycotoxins are readily absorbed by various modes, including the topical, oral, and inhalational routes [87]. Intestinal epithelial cells newly identified as an important target for trichothecenes, which affect the network of tight junctions and thus lead to impaired intestinal barrier function, impairing nutrient transport, the immune system, and increased risk of transmission of pathogens and antigens from the intestinal lumen to surrounding tissues, increased the possibility of allergic reactions in humans [88].

12. Conclusion

This review showed the main dangerous effect of mycotoxins on public health and the occurrence of dangerous diseases such as cancer and mutations by some of them such as aflatoxins. In addition to its transmission through the food chains, it was also found that there is the ability of different species of fungi to secrete mycotoxins at a wide range of different environmental factors, in addition to their occurrence in the pre- and postharvest stages and during poor storage conditions and marketing to the consumer (human and animal). In view of the seriousness and importance of this topic, more light should be shed on mycotoxins and their occurrence in many agricultural, food, and feed products, especially in developing countries, should be shed light on the lack of accurate systems and programs that reveal this. And since the effect on the public health of mycotoxins does not appear quickly until after long periods, they really represent the silent or slow death of humans and animals, modern strategies, means and methods must be followed to prevent the occurrence of mycotoxins, especially in the pre- and postharvest stages and in the store, represented by genetic, agricultural, biological, chemical, and physical methods.

Author details

Azhar A. Alhaddad
Department of Plant Protection, College of Agriculture, University of Basrah, Iraq

*Address all correspondence to: azhar1982ha@gmail.com;
azhar.hassan@uobasrah.edu.iq

References

[1] Peraica M, Radica B, Lucica A, Pavlovic M. Toxic effects of mycotoxins in humans. Bulletin of the World Health Organization. 1999;**77**(9):754-766

[2] Tola M, Kebede B. Occurrence, importance and control of mycotoxins: A review. Cogent Food Agriculture. 2016;**2**:1-12

[3] Bennett JW. Mycotoxins, mycotoxicoses, mycotoxicology and Mycopathologia. Mycopathologia. 1987;**100**:3-5

[4] Rudolf K, John L, Richard R, Schuhmacher A, Slate B, Thomas W. Romer Labs Guide to Mycotoxins. Leicestershire, England: Anytime Publishing Services; 2012. p. 127

[5] Pittet AC. Natural occurrence of mycotoxins in foods and feeds: An update review. Revista de Medicina Veterinaria. 1998;**6**:479-492

[6] FAO/WHO. JECFA Safety evaluation of certain contaminants in food. WHO Food Additive Series. 2011;**63**:1-791

[7] Bhat R, Rai RV, Karim AA. Mycotoxins in food and feed: Present status and future concerns. Comprehensive Reviews in Food Science and Food Safety. 2010;**9**(1):57-81

[8] Richard JL. Some major mycotoxins and their mycotoxicoses an overview. International Journal of Food Microbiology. 2007;**119**(1-2):3-10

[9] Filtenborg O, Frisvad JC, Thrane U. Moulds in food spoilage. International Journal of Food Microbiology. 1996;**33**(1):85-102

[10] Capriotti AL, Caruso G, Cavaliere C, Foglia P, Samperi R, Laganà A. Multiclass mycotoxin analysis in food, environmental and biological matrices with chromatography/mass spectrometry. Mass Spectrometry Reviews. 2012;**31**(4):466-503

[11] Karlovsky P, Suman M, Berthiller F, De Meester J, Eisenbrand G, Perrin I, et al. Impact of food processing and detoxification treatments on mycotoxin contamination. Mycotoxin Research. 2016;**32**(4):179-205

[12] Piotrowska M, Śliżewska K, Biernasiak J. Mycotoxins in cereal and soybean-based food and feed. In: Chapter 8. Soybean: Pest Resistance. Intech; 2018. pp. 185-230

[13] Miller JD. Fungi and mycotoxins in grain: Implications for stored product research. Journal of Stored Products Research. 1995;**31**:1-16

[14] Olsen M, Johnsson P, Möller T, Paladino R, Lindblad M. Aspergillus nomius, an important aflatoxin producer in Brazil nuts? World Mycotoxin Journal. 2008;**1**(2):123-126

[15] Pitt JI, Hocking AD. Fungi and Food Spoilage. 3rd ed. New York: Springer; 2009. p. 503

[16] Pitt JI, Miscamble BF. Water relations of Aspergillus flavus and closely related species. Journal of Food Protection. 1995;**58**:86-90

[17] Wheeler KA, Hurdman BF, Pitt JI. Influence of pH on the growth of some toxigenic species of Aspergillus, Penicillium and Fusarium. International Journal of Food Microbiology. 1991;**12**:141-149

[18] Bazioli JM, Amaral LDS, Fill TP, Rodrigues-Filho E. Insights into

Penicillium brasilianum secondary metabolism and its biotechnological potential. Molecules. 2017;**22**(6):858-880

[19] Cho HS, Hong SB, Go SJ. First report of *Penicillium brasilianum* and *P. daleae* isolated from soil in Korea. Mycobiology. 2005;**33**(2):113-117

[20] Houbraken J, Kocsubé S, Visagie CM, Yilmaz N, Wang XC, Meijer M, et al. Classification of Aspergillus, Penicillium, Talaromyces and related genera (Eurotiales): An overview of families, genera, subgenera, sections, series and species. Studies in Mycology. 2020;**95**:5-169

[21] González MC, Lull C, Moya P, Ayala I, Primo J, Primo Yúfera E. Insecticidal activity of penitrems, including penitrem G, a new member of the family isolated from Penicillium crustosum. Journal of Agricultural and Food Chemistry. 2003;**51**:2156-2160

[22] Nicoletti R, Lopez-Gresa MP, Manzo E, Carella A, Ciavatta ML. Production and fungitoxic activity of Sch 642305, a secondary metabolite of Penicillium canescens. Mycopathologia. 2007;**163**:301-395

[23] Dean R, Van Kan JAL, Pretorius ZA, Hammond-Kosack KE, Di Pietro A, Spanu PD, et al. The top 10 fungal pathogens in molecular plant pathology: Top 10 fungal pathogens. Molecular Plant Pathology. 2012;**13**(4):414-430

[24] Lin B, Bozorgmagham A, Ross SD, Schmale DG. Small fluctuations in the recovery of fusaria across consecutive sampling intervals with unmanned aircraft 100 m above ground level. Aerobiologia. 2013;**29**:45-54

[25] Pal N, Kumar A, Malannavar AB. Effect of temperature and pH levels on the growth and sporulation of Fusarium oxysporum f.sp. lini causing linseed wilt. International Journal of Chemical Studies. 2019;**7**(3):4494-4497

[26] Aoki T, O'Donnell K, Geiser DM. Systematics of key phytopathogenic Fusarium species: Current status and future challenges. Journal of General Plant Pathology. 2014;**80**(3):189-201

[27] Bai GH, Desjardins AE, Plattner RD. Deoxynivalenol-nonproducing Fusarium graminearum causes initial infection, but does not cause disease spread in wheat spikes. Mycopathologia. 2002;**153**:91-98

[28] Desmond OJ, Manners JM, Stephens AE, Maclean DJ, Schenk PM, Gradiner DM, et al. The Fusarium mycotoxins deoxynivalenol elicits hydrogen peroxide production, programmed cell death and defence responses in wheat. Molecular Plant Pathology. 2008;**9**(4):435-445

[29] Krska R, Josephs R. The state-of-the-art in the analysis of estrogenic mycotoxins in cereals. Fresenius' Journal of Analytical Chemistry. 2001;**369**(6):469-476

[30] Brown DW, Lee SH, Kim LH, Ryu JG, Lee S, Seo Y, et al. Identification of a 12-gene fusaric acid biosynthetic gene cluster in Fusarium species through comparative and functional genomics. Molecular Plant-Microbe Interactions. 2015;**28**(3):319-332

[31] Jestoi M. Emerging Fusarium-mycotoxins fusaproliferin, beauvericin, enniatins, and moniliformina : A review. Critical Reviews Food Science and Nutrition. 2008;**48**(1):21-49

[32] Rudolf K, John LR, Rainer S, Andrew BS, Thomas BW. Romer Labs Guide to Mycotoxins. 4th ed. Leicestershire, England: Anytime Publishing Services; 2015. p. 114

[33] Shaw CI. Chemical residues, food additives and natural toxicants in food, the cocktail effect. International Journal of Food Science and Technology. 2014;**49**:2149-2157

[34] Phillips TD, Lemke SL, Grant PG. Characterization of claybased enterosorbents for the prevention of aflatoxicosis BT—mycotoxins and food SAfety. Advances in Experimental Medicine and Biology. 2002;**51**:61-99

[35] Mariya K, Zakhar C, Irina S, Ilya A. Stability of mycotoxins in individual stock and multi-analyte standard solutions. Toxins. 2020;**12**(94):1-22

[36] Winnie P, Pui L, Sabran M. Mycotoxin: Its impact on gut health and microbiota. Frontiers in Cellular and Infection Microbiology. 2018;**8**:1-17

[37] Mowaffaq AA, Yasser MT, Khirun BM, Doblin AS. Effects of different mycotoxins on humans, cell genome and their involvement in cancer (review). Oncology Reports. 2017;**37**:1321-1336

[38] Alshannaq A, Yu JH. Occurrence, toxicity, and analysis of major mycotoxins in food. International Journal of Environmental Research and Public Health. 2017;**14**(632):1-20

[39] Fountain JC, Khera P, Yang L, Nayak SN, Scully BT, Lee RD, et al. Resistance to Aspergillus flavus in maize and peanut: Molecular biology, breeding, environmental stress, and future perspectives. Crop Journal. 2015;**3**:229-237

[40] Varzakas T. Quality and safety aspects of cereals (Wheat) and their products. Critical Reviews in Food Science and Nutrition. 2016;**56**:2495-2510

[41] Fernandes TH, Ferrão J, Bell V, Chabite IT. Mycotoxins, food and health. Journal of Nutrition Health Food Sciences. 2017;**5**(7):1-10

[42] Schmidt-Heydt M, Abdel-Hadi A, Magan N, Geisen R. Complex regulation of the aflatoxin biosynthesis gene cluster of Aspergillus flavus in relation to various combinations of water activity and temperature. International Journal of Food Microbiology. 2009;**135**:231-237

[43] Maria EB, Francisco CO, Fábio EF, Maria IF, Davide R. Mycotoxins and their effects on human and animal health. Food Control. 2014;**36**:159-165

[44] Lee HJ, Ryu D. Worldwide occurrence of mycotoxins in cereals and cereal-derived food products: Public health perspectives of their co-occurrence. Journal of Agricultural and Food Chemistry. 2017;**65**:7034-7051

[45] Marin S, Ramos AJ, Cano-Sancho G, Sanchis V. Mycotoxins: Occurrence, toxicology, and exposure assessment. Food and Chemical Toxicology. 2013;**60**:218-237

[46] WHO (World Health Organization). New IARC report urges action against widespread mycotoxin contamination in developing countries. IARC WHO Press Release. 2016;**9**:2015-2016

[47] Bokhari FM. Implications of fungal infections and mycotoxins in camel diseases in Saudi Arabia. Saudi Journal of Biological Science. 2010;**17**:73-81

[48] Wild CP, Hall AJ. Primary prevention of hepatocellular carcinoma in developing countries. Mutation Research. 2000;**462**:381-393

[49] Dusanne T. Importance of aflatoxins. KMITL. 2002;**2**(1):38-54

[50] Wu F, Stacy SL, Kensler TW. Global risk assessment of aflatoxins in maize

and peanuts: Are regulatory standards adequately protective? Toxicological Sciences. 2013;**135**:251-259

[51] Vanhoutte I, Audenaert K, De Gelder L. Biodegradation of mycotoxins: Tales from known and unexplored worlds. Frontiers in Microbiology. 2016;**7**(561):1-20

[52] Benkerroum N. Mycotoxins in dairy products: A review. International Dairy Journal. 2016;**62**:63-75

[53] Sirhan AY, Tan GH, Al-Shunnaq A, Abdulra'uf L, Wong RC. Quenchers-HPLC method for aflatoxin detection of domestic and imported food in Jordan. Journal of Liquid Chromatography Related Technology. 2014;**37**:321-342

[54] Tomlins K, Jewers K, Coker R. Evaluation of non-polar bonded-phases for the clean-up of maize extracts prior to aflatoxin assay by HPTLC. Chromatographia. 1989;**27**:67-70

[55] Gotah A, Whang K, Garcia C. Determination of aflatoxins in rice using quechers and fluorescence HPLC. Chemistry & Chemical Engineering, Biotechnology, Food Industry. 2018;**19**(2):133-141

[56] Haque M, Wang Y, Shen Z, Li X, Saleemi M, He C. Mycotoxin contamination and control strategy in human, domestic animal and poultry: A review. Journal Pre-proof. 2020;**142**:1-27

[57] Schaafsma AW, Hooker DC. Climatic to predict occurrence of Fusarium toxins in wheat and models maize. International Journal of Food Microbiology. 2007;**119**:116-125

[58] Cole RA, Jarvis BB, Schweikert MA. Handbook of Secondary Metabolites. New York: Academic Press; 2003. pp. 199-560

[59] EFSA (European Food Safety Authority). Scientific Opinion on the risks for animal and public health related to the presence of T-2 and HT-2 toxin in food and feed. EFSA Journal. 2011a;**9**(12):2481

[60] EFSA (European Food Safety Authority). Scientific opinion on the risks for animal and public health related to the presence of T-2 and HT-2 toxin in food and feed. EFSA Journal. 2011b;**9**(12):2481-2668

[61] Mc Cormick SP, Stanley AM, Stover NA, Alexander NJ. Trichothecenes: From simple to complex mycotoxins. Toxins. 2011;**3**:802-814

[62] Chen P, Xiang B, Shi H, Yu P, Song Y, Li S. Recent advances on type A trichothecenes in food and feed: Analysis, prevalence, toxicity, and decontamination techniques. Food Control. 2020;**118**:107-371

[63] Agriopoulou S, Stamatelopoulou E, Varzakas T. Advances in occurrence, importance, and mycotoxin control strategies: Prevention and detoxification in foods. Food. 2020;**9**(137):1-48

[64] Shank RA, Foroud NA, Hazendonk P, Eudes F, Blackwell BA. Current and future experimental strategies for structural analysis of trichothecene mycotoxins—A prospectus. Toxins. 2011;**3**:1518-1553

[65] Ji F, He D, Olaniran AO, Mokoena MP, Xu J, Shi J. Occurrence, toxicity, production and detection of Fusarium mycotoxin: A review. Food Production, Processing and Nutrition. 2019;**1**(6):1-14

[66] Frisvad JC. A critical review of producers of small lactone mycotoxins: Patulin, penicillic acid and moniliformin. World Mycotoxin Journal. 2018;**11**(1):73-100

[67] Puel O, Galtier P, Oswald IP. Biosynthesis and toxicological effects of patulin. Toxins. 2010;**2**:613-631

[68] Sant'Ana AS, Simas RC, Almeida CAA, Cabral EC, Rauber RH, Mallmann CA. Influence of package, type of apple juice and temperature on the production of patulin by Byssochlamys nivea and Byssochlamys fulva. International Journal of Food Microbiology. 2010;**142**:156-163

[69] Erdoğan A, Ghimire D, Gürses M, Çetin B, Baran A. Patulin contamination in fruit juices and its control measures. European Journal of Science and Technology. 2018;**14**:39-48

[70] Forouzan S, Madadlou A. Incidence of patulin in apple juices produced in west Azerbayjan Province, Iran. Journal of Agricultural Science and Technology. 2014;**16**:1613-1622

[71] Vidal A, Ouhibi S, Ghali R, Hedhili A, De Saeger S, De Boevre M. The mycotoxin patulin: An updated short review on occurrence, toxicity and analytical challenges. Food and Chemical Toxicology. 2019;**129**:249-256

[72] Leung MCK, Diaz-Llano G, Smith TK. Mycotoxins in pet food: A review on worldwide prevalence and preventative strategies. Journal of Agricultural and Food Chemistry. 2006;**54**:9623-9635

[73] Gajecka M, Stopa E, Tarasiuk M, Zielonka Ł, Gajecki M. The expression of type-1 and type-2 nitric oxide synthase in selected tissues of the gastrointestinal tract during mixed mycotoxicosis. Toxins. 2013;**5**:2281-2292

[74] Hernández-Martínez R, Navarro-Blasco I. Aflatoxin levels and exposure assessment of Spanish infant cereals. Food Additives & Contaminants. Part B, Surveillance. 2010;**3**:275-288

[75] IARC (International Agency for Research on Cancer). Some naturally occurring substances: Food items and constituents, heterocyclic aromatic amines and mycotoxins. IARC Monographs on the Evaluation of Carcinogenic Risks to Humans. 1993;**56**:1-609

[76] Strosnider H, Azziz-Baumgartner E, Banziger M, Bhat RV, Breiman R, Brune MN, et al. Workgroup report: Public health strategies for reducing aflatoxin exposure in developing countries. Environmental Health Perspectives. 2006;**114**(12):1898-1903

[77] Zinedine A, Mañes J. Occurrence and legislation of mycotoxins in food and feed from Morocco. Food Control. 2009;**20**:334-344

[78] Hall AJ, Wild CP. Liver cancer in low and middle income countries. British Medical Journal. 2003;**326**(7379):994-995

[79] Williams JH, Phillips TD, Jolly PE, Stiles JK, Jolly CM, Aggarwal D. Human aflatoxicosis in developing countries: A review of toxicology, exposure, potential health consequences, and interventions. The American Journal of Clinical Nutrition. 2004;**80**(5):1106-1122

[80] Bennett JW, Klich M. Mycotoxins. Clinical Microbiology Reviews. 2003;**16**(3):497-516

[81] FDA. GUIDANCE DOCUMENT/ Guidance for Industry: Action Levels for Poisonous or Deleterious Substances in Human Food and Animal Feed2013. pp. 1-20. Available from: https:// www.regulations.gov/document/ FDA-2020-D-1956-0001

[82] Zhu M, Cen Y, Ye W, Li S, Zhang W. Recent advances on macrocyclic trichothecenes, their bioactivities and biosynthetic pathway. Toxins. 2020;**12**(417):1-16

[83] Pinton P, Oswald IP. Effect of deoxynivalenol and other Type B trichothecenes on the intestine: A review. Toxins. 2014;**6**:1615-1643

[84] Polak-Sliwinska M, Paszczyk B. Trichothecenes in food and feed, relevance to human and animal health and methods of detection: A systematic review. Molecules. 2021;**26**(454):1-22

[85] Tericiolo C, Maresca M, Pinton P, Oswald IP. Role of satiety hormones in anorexia induction by Trichothecene mycotoxins. Food Chemical Toxicology. 2018;**121**:701-714

[86] Li M, Cuff CF, Pestka J. Modulation of murine host response to enteric reovirus infection by the trichothecene deoxynivalenol. Toxicology Sciences. 2005;**87**(1):134-145

[87] Wu Q, Wu W, Tanos C, Franca C, Jacevic V, Wang X, et al. Immune evasion, a potential mechanism of trichothecenes: New insights into negative immune regulations. International Journal of Molecular Sciences. 2018;**19**(3307):1-4

[88] Akbari P, Braber S, Varasteh S, Alizadeh A, Garssen J, Fink-Gremmels J. The intestinal barrier as an emerging target in the toxicological assessment of mycotoxins. Archives of Toxicology. 2016;**91**:1007-1029

Section 3

Mycotoxins in Feed

Chapter 4

Animal Feeds Mycotoxins and Risk Management

Zacharia Waithaka Ng'ang'a and Eric Niyonshuti

Abstract

The demand for livestock products is the main factor affecting the demand for livestock feeds worldwide. However, animal feed safety has gradually become more important, with mycotoxins representing one of the most significant hazards. Mycotoxins are toxic secondary metabolites produced naturally by fungi that grow on various agriculture commodities. Aflatoxin, fumonisin, ochratoxin, trichothecene, and zearalenone are the more prevalent mycotoxins in animal feeds. Some of mycotoxins impacts include; loss of animal and human health, reduced animal productivity, increased veterinary service costs, feed disposal and increased research costs which enhance the importance of mycotoxins detoxification. Contamination of feeds may occur both during pre-harvest and post-harvest. The purpose of this chapter is to review the most prevalent mycotoxins in animal feeds, reveal the origin of mycotoxins contamination and the possible risks they pose to feeds and livestock. This chapter also gives an overview of the most important factors that influence mold growth and mycotoxin production as well as the economic impacts of mycotoxins. To the end of this chapter, mycotoxins preventive methods, both preharvest and postharvest, are well discussed.

Keywords: mycotoxins, mold, animal, nutrition, prevention, detoxification

1. Introduction

The demand for livestock products is the main factor affecting the demand for livestock feeds worldwide. The world-wide demand for animal feed is expected to increase as a result of the global demand for animal sourced food which is expected to increase due to growth of the world population. The United Nations Food and Agriculture Organization (FAO) estimates that food demand will increase by 60% by 2050, and animal protein production will increase by 1.7% per year between 2010 and 2050, with meat production expected to increase by nearly 70%, aquaculture by 90%, and dairy by 55% [1, 2]. However, animal feed safety has gradually become more important, with mycotoxins representing one of the most significant hazards [3]. Mycotoxins are secondary metabolites produced naturally by filamentous fungi, which are considered toxic substances when present in food for humans and feed for animals [4]. They are small and quite stable molecules which are extremely difficult to remove or eradicate, and which enter the feed chain while keeping their toxic properties.

More than 500 mycotoxins have been identified, the majority of which have been either regulated or tested [5]. These chemically different mycotoxins formed by more than 350 fungal species and causing diseases to living organisms have been researched [6] but only a few have been extensively researched and even fewer have good methods of analysis [7]. The primary classes of mycotoxins are aflatoxins (B1, B2, G1, G2) of which aflatoxin B1 (AFB1) is the most prevalent, zearalenone (ZEA), trichothecenes such as deoxynivalenol (DON) and T-2 toxin (T-2), fumonisins (FUM: FB1, FB2, FB3) and ochratoxin A (OTA) [8]. With regard to animal feed, aflatoxins, fumonisins, ochratoxins, trichothecenes, and zearalenone are the more prevalent ones hazards [3]. The majority of mycotoxins in these groups are produced by three fungal genera: Aspergillus, Penicillium and Fusarium [9]. Many species of these fungi produce mycotoxins in animal feedstuffs. Because a given mold species can produce many types of mycotoxins in a single food item, multiple contaminations are possible. Multiple varieties of mycotoxins can also be discovered in the same feed if it contains a variety of contaminated products or raw materials. Several studies and surveys that revealed concurrent contamination were mentioned in a review on mycotoxins in the human food chain by Galvano et al. There is therefore a risk of simultaneous contamination in animal feed since raw cereals can also be employed as raw materials in animal feed preparation [10].

Mycotoxin contamination usually occur in the field as well as during processing and storage of feed products as long as the conditions allow fungal colonization with moisture content and ambient temperature being the key determinants of this mycotoxin production [11]. Mold growth in feeds is undesirable because they secrete toxins which impair with animal health and productivity [12]. Direct consequences of consumption of mycotoxins-contaminated livestock feed include reduced feed intake, feed refusal, poor feed conversion, diminished body weight gain, increased disease incidence, and reduced reproductive capacities [13]. Furthermore, mycotoxins could potentially impose large costs on the economy [14]. The addition of adsorbents to feeds is the most widely applied way of protecting animals against mycotoxins.

However, it is quite relevant to understand possible sources of mycotoxins that contaminate animal feeds and the various available preventive methods that can be explored. This review is intended to explore and provide information about most prevalent mycotoxins in animal feeds. The review also highlights the origin of mycotoxins in feeds, the possible risks they pose to feeds and livestock production in general. To the end of this article, mycotoxins preventive methods and mycotoxins risk management methods both before and after harvesting animal feeds are well discussed.

2. Mycotoxins and fungi classification

Mycotoxins are toxic secondary metabolites produced naturally by filamentous fungi that grow on various agriculture commodities [4, 15]. The main factors influencing fungi growth and mycotoxin production are temperature and moisture [14]. The mycotoxin contamination can occur during pre-harvest and post-harvest, this is why researchers have divided fungal species into two main groups: field fungi and storage fungi [12].

Field fungi invade the seeds while the crop is still in the field and require high moisture conditions (20–21%). These include species of *Fusarium*, *Alternaria*, *Cladosporium*, *Diplodia*, *Gibberella* and *Helminthosporium*. On the other hand, storage fungi are those that invade grain or seeds during storage and require less moisture than field fungi (13–18%). Storage fungi include species of *Aspergillus* and *Penicillium* [12]. It's important to remember that not all fungal growth results in the production of mycotoxins, and that the detection of fungi does not always suggest the presence of mycotoxins.

Mycotoxigenic species may be further classified based on their geographical prevalence. *Aspergillus flavus*, *A. parasiticus* and *A. ochraceus* readily proliferate under warm and humid conditions, while *Penicillium expansum* and *P. verrucosum* are essentially temperate fungi. Fusarium fungi are more ubiquitous, but toxigenic species from this genus are less likely to be associated with cereals contamination from warm countries [11].

Mycotoxins are classified according to their chemical structures and biological activities as; carcinogenic (e.g. aflatoxin B1, ochratoxin A, fumonisin B1), oestrogenic (zearalenone), neurotoxic (fumonisin B1), nephrotoxic (ochratoxins, citrinin, oosporein), dermonecrotic (trichothecenes) and immunosuppressive (aflatoxin B1, ochratoxin A, and T-2 toxin) [16].

3. Major mycotoxins in animal feeds and toxicity

According to different reports, more than 400 mycotoxins have been identified. Mycotoxins can occur under natural conditions in animal feeds. Most mycotoxins of concern in the area of animal nutrition are produced by three genera of fungi, namely, Aspergillus, Penicillium, and Fusarium (**Table 1**) [19]. Biomin, a feed additive manufacturer, conducted a two-year assessment to assess the incidence of mycotoxins in feed and feed raw materials in several of the key animal production locations. AFB1, OTA, DON, T2 toxin, ZEA, and fumonisins were determined in a total of 2753 assays on 1507 samples collected from European and Mediterranean markets. Mycotoxins were found in 52% of these samples, demonstrating that the prevalence of mycotoxins in animal feed is relatively significant [20].

3.1 Aflatoxin

Aflatoxins are produced by strains of *Aspergillus flavus* and *A. Parasiticus* and they are a prominent cause of disease in animals. Naturally occurring aflatoxins are B1, B2, G1 and G2. Aflatoxin B1 is the most prevalent of the aflatoxins and occur in a couple of important animal feeds. It is one of the most potent hepatocarcinogens and causes

Mycotoxin	Molds/fungal species
Aflatoxin	*Aspergillus flavus, A. parasiticus*
Deoxynivalenol	*Fusarium culmorum, F. graminearum, F. sporotrichioides*
Ochratoxin A	*A. ochraceus, A. Alliaceus, A. melleus, A. ostianus, A. sulphureus, Penicillium viridicatum, P. palitans, P. commune, P. variabile, P. cyclopium, P. verrucosum, P. purescens*
T-2 toxin	*F. acuminatum, F. equiseti, F. poae, F. semitectum, F. sporotrichioides*
Zearalenone	*F. culmorum, F. graminearum, F. sambucinum, F. semitectum, F. sporotrichioides*
Fumonisins	*F. proliferatum, F. verticillioides*

Table 1.
Some key species of molds producing some of the most important mycotoxins in animal husbandry [17, 18].

acute hepatotoxicity as well as growth retardation in animals. Aflatoxin contaminates most agricultural commodities. The highest levels of contamination have been recorded in groundnuts, tree nuts, other oilseeds and corn. Corn, cottonseed, and peanuts are some of the most important sources of aflatoxin in animal feeds [21]. Small cereal grains (barley, oats, and wheat) are also occasionally colonized by the causative molds, which produce low to moderate quantities of aflatoxin. Soybeans do not support significant levels of aflatoxin B1 production [22].

Worldwide aflatoxins have been reported to be prevalent in both feedstuffs and finished feeds [23]. Aflatoxin is posing a dangerous problem for animal industry and human health [24]. Concerning livestock health, Aflatoxins cause acute death to chronic disease. Chronic aflatoxins poisoning causes a wide range of symptoms that aren't always visible clinically; a slow rate of growth in young animals is a sensitive clinical indicator of chronic aflatoxicosis. Aflatoxicosis is characterized by a decrease in total production, greater vulnerability to stressors, and clinical manifestations such as gastrointestinal problems [3]. Long-term consumption of aflatoxin contaminated feeds results in negative effects on the liver (primary target organ), such as hepatic cell and tissue injury, as well as gross abnormalities [25, 26].

3.2 Ochratoxin

Ochratoxin is a dangerous mycotoxin, produced by Aspergillus species in warmer climates and Penicillium species in cold areas. Ochratoxin contaminates various raw agricultural commodities and has dangerous effects on animals and humans [27]. Ochratoxin predominantly affects the kidneys of all animal species, but it can also harm the liver at high concentrations. Because of its strong protein affinity, especially for albumin, ochratoxin A (OTA), a primary ochratoxin, accumulates in animal tissues. OTA has been proved to be a potent nephrotoxic, immunotoxic, neurotoxic, hepatotoxic, and teratogenic compound. The intake of feed contaminated with OTA affects animal health and productivity [28]. The kidneys are the most affected by OTA-acute toxicity, and pigs have the highest susceptibility, developing nephropathy following exposure [29]. Many animal studies, including chick, quail, rabbit, hamster, rat, and mouse research, indicated teratogenic effects, with craniofacial deformities and lower birth weight being the most prevalent [30, 31]. The most relevant effects of ochratoxins in animal cells are the inhibition of protein synthesis, lipid peroxidation, DNA damage and oxidoreductive stress [32].

3.3 Zearalenone

Zearalenone is one of the well-known mycotoxins produced by Fusarium mold species [33]. The fungi that produce zearalenone are distributed worldwide, particularly in cereal grains and derived products [34]. Zearalenone is a stable compound during storage and can resist high temperature during processing of food [35]. Furthermore, it was observed that during feed processing (e.g., milling, extrusion, storage and heating) zearalenone was not decomposed [36]. It can be found in all products intended for animal feeding [33]. It is recommended that the overall amount of zearalenone in the diet should not exceed 250 ppb [37]. It has been concluded that zearalenone interacts with estrogen receptors and causes an oestrogenic response in animals [38]. Among its estrogenic effects includes decreased fertility, increased embryo lethal resorptions, reduced litter size, change in serum levels of progesterone and teratogenic effects in pigs and sheep [35].

At higher doses, zearalenone interferes with conception, ovulation, implantation, fetal development and the viability of newborn animals [37]. Large doses of zearalenone toxin are associated with abortions in dairy cattle as well as reduced feed intake, decreased milk production, vaginitis, increase vaginal secretions, poor reproductive performance and mammary gland enlargement in heifers. Swine have been shown to be the most sensitive to zearalenone among farm animals; some consequences in pigs include swelling of the vulva and mammary glands, stillbirth, prolonged estrus intervals, vulvovaginitis, vaginal and/or rectal prolapse, ovarian atrophy, disrupted conception, abortion and infertility [39–41]. In male pigs, zearalenone induces feminization, decreases spermatogenesis, testicular weight, decreases libido, and decreases testosterone levels [37].

3.4 Fumonisins

Fumonisins are neurotoxic and possible carcinogens. Fumonisins are hydrophilic, unlike other known mycotoxins, which are soluble in organic solvents, making them challenging to study. Different fumonisins have been previously identified (FA1, FA2, FB1, FB2, FB3 and FB4) [42]. Fumonisins causes liver and kidney damage, decreases weight gains, impairs immune function and increases mortality rates in most animals. FB1 and FB2 were isolated from *F. moniliforme* cultures and were found to promote cancer in rats [42]. Fumonisins occur naturally in corn, and they have been linked with equine leukoencephalomalacia which results in softening of white tissue in the brain [41]. Interference with the enzyme N-acyltransferase, which is involved in sphingolipid metabolism, is the principal mechanism of fumonisins toxicity. This mainly results in the disruption of processes involved in liver functioning as well as affecting other biological functions such as protein metabolism and the urea cycle [41, 43].

3.5 Trichothecenes

Trichothecenes are produced mainly, but not only, by Fusarium species. With a basis on the chemical structure, more toxic but less prevalent type A trichothecenes (T-2) and widely occurring type B trichothecenes (deoxynivalenol, DON) are well defined [44]. Trichothecenes are mostly found in cereals, commercial cattle feed and mixed feeds. They affect livestock animals, pets and humans [14]. Trichothecenes can be easily absorbed via the skin and gastrointestinal tract [5]. Ingestion of feeds contaminated by trichothecenes results in decreased feed intake and weight gain, bloody diarrhea, hemorrhaging, oral lesions, low productivity, immunosuppression, abortion, and sometimes death [3, 45].

Trichothecenes have several action mechanisms, including DNA, RNA, and protein synthesis inhibition, neurotransmitter alterations, lipid peroxidation, apoptosis, mitochondrial function inhibition, and cytokine activation [46, 47]. Through microbial degradation of trichothecenes in the gastrointestinal system, monogastric animals, particularly young pigs, are very sensitive, although poultry and ruminants appear to be less sensitive to some trichothecenes [46]. Because of inadequate absorption following oral exposure, extensive metabolism, and rapid removal from the body, poultry have a higher tolerance to trichothecenes [48, 49].

3.5.1 T-2 toxin

T-2 is the most lethal of the trichothecene mycotoxins, and its toxicity in animals varies depending on age, dosage, and species. The T-2 toxin, which is mostly produced by *Fusarium tricinctum*, was the first trichothecene to be discovered as a naturally occurring grain contaminant in the United States, where it was linked to a deadly toxicosis in dairy animals fed moldy corn [50]. T-2 toxin was found to inhibit protein and DNA synthesis and weaken cellular immune responses in animals [51]. T-2 toxin has been linked to feed refusal, output losses, diarrhea, intestinal hemorrhages, and death in dairy cattle. In poultry, the T-2 toxin has been linked to oral and intestinal lesions, as well as immune system impairment, hematopoietic system destruction, decreased egg production, thinning of eggshells, feed refusal, weight loss, altered feather patterns, and incorrect wing positioning [52, 53]. Cells that divide rapidly are more vulnerable to T-2 toxin thereby explaining why the immune system and the gastrointestinal tract are two of T-2's primary targets. Carcinogenesis, immunological depression, neurotransmitter abnormalities, weight loss, growth retardation, oral lesions, diarrhea, and vomiting are among indications of chronic and acute T-2 toxicity in animals [5, 47, 54].

3.5.2 Deoxynivalenol (vomitoxin)

Deoxynivalenol (DON) is one of the most frequently detected trichothecenes in grains [55] and the most common producing species of deoxynivalenol (DON) is *F. graminearum* [56]. DON is stable and it can survive processing, milling. Therefore, it easily occurs in feeds prepared from contaminated corn and wheat.

Swine are the most vulnerable of all livestock species to deoxynivalenol (DON) toxicity. The main symptoms for DON are vomiting (hence known as "vomitoxin"), feed refusal, skin damage and hemorrhage especially in swine [44]. DON has been associated with reduced milk production in dairy cattle, reproductive performance inhibition and immune function inhibition in several animal species [56]. Low intakes of DON causes nausea, diarrhea, gastrointestinal tract lesions, decreased nutritional efficiency, and weight loss in animals while higher doses of DON intake induces vomiting and feed refusal with severe reduction in weight, severe damage in the hematopoietic systems and immune dysregulation [57–59]. Dogs and cats can be affected as well, and sensitivity to DON mainly vary with gender and age [5, 60].

4. Factors influencing mold growth and mycotoxin production

The production of mycotoxins requires molds growth [18]. The production of these compounds, especially in grains, is highly dependent on environmental factors pre and/or postharvest (**Table 2**) [61]. Temperature, relative humidity strains of toxigenic organisms and occurrence of competitive growth are the most factors responsible for mold outbreaks in the field [62]. Temperature, water activity, and oxygen are the most significant elements for growth and mycotoxin generation, aside from the presence of nutrients. Physical and chemical features of substrates affect their ability to support fungal growth. Physical qualities include water activity, oxygen availability, and surface area, while chemical characteristics include carbohydrates, lipids, protein, trace elements, and amino acid composition [63].

According to [64], a minimum water activity of 0.70 will sustain growth of storage molds, though for field molds that produce mycotoxins water activity should be above 0.85. Most fungi require the relative humidity to be above 70% for them to develop. At a moisture level of 14–15%, in equilibrium with a relative humidity of 70–75%, *Aspergillus glaucus* will develop and thrive on cereals, pulses, pellets, and defatted

Mycotoxin	Temperature (°C)	Water activity
Aflatoxin	33	0.99
Ochratoxin	25–30	0.98
Fumonisin	15–30	0.9–0.995
Zearalenone	25	0.96
Deoxynivalenol	26–30	0.995

Table 2.
The optimum temperature and water activity for mycotoxins production in grains [61].

oilseed meals [65]. At the same relative humidity, the moisture levels of the whole oilseeds such as rapeseed, sunflower, or flax will be only 6–7%, but the fungi will still develop.

Many researchers have reported that pre-harvest fungal invasion is influenced by in-field damage caused by insects, birds, rodents, husbandry practices and adverse weather. Stress caused by drought, nutrient deficiency and untimely or excessive fertilizer application may also predispose towards fungal establishment. Airborne fungal spores can easily infect cracked grain, whereas soil-borne spores can easily infect pods and cobs of crops that fall to the ground. Mold is encouraged and fungal infection is favored by repeated planting of the same crop in the same field, poor harvest handling, poor storage, and post-harvest pest attack.

5. Overview of mycotoxin effects in animals

Intake levels, duration of exposure, toxin species, modes of action, metabolism, and defense systems all influence the harmful effect of mycotoxin ingestion in animals. The presence of multiple mycotoxins in feed probably have at least an additive, if not synergistic, effect. In animals, mycotoxins have a wide range of biological consequences, including liver and kidney damage, neurological effects, immune-suppressive effects, carcinogenic, estrogenic and teratogenic effects, to mention a few. Carcinogenic examples of mycotoxins include AFB1, OTA, and FB1. When mold and mycotoxins are present together, it can lead to infection risk, as well as reproductive issues. Animals that consume mycotoxin-contaminated feed may experience appetite loss, reduced feed efficiency, immunosuppression (leading to increased disease incidence), poor weight gain, and mortality [7, 39, 66].

It should be noted that toxicity may vary considerably within a structural group of mycotoxins and that the danger may not always be due to the toxin itself but to its metabolites. Chronic intoxication can adversely affect animal health, leading to problems with reproduction, increased susceptibility to infectious diseases, and altered performance. According to a review by [5], mycotoxins exhibit their cellular/molecular effects via several mechanisms including metabolic enzyme inhibition, ribosomal binding, DNA effects, protein interaction, ionophore activity, effects on hormones, epigenetic properties, necrosis and apoptosis, RNA polymerase effects, and mitochondrial interactions. Mycotoxins have varied impacts on various organ systems and cellular pathways. Aflatoxin, ochratoxin, and T-2 toxin, for example, all inhibit protein synthesis, but in distinct ways: aflatoxin binds to both RNA and DNA and stops transcription, T-2 toxin inhibits translation initiation, and ochratoxin inhibits phenylalanine-t RNA synthetase and hence translation [67].

Mycotoxins are capable of inducing both acute and chronic effects. The effects observed are often related to dose levels and duration of exposure. Acute primary mycotoxicosis occurs if high to moderate amounts of mycotoxins are consumed. Specific, overt, acute episodes of disease ensue, which include hepatitis, hemorrhage, nephritis, necrosis of oral and enteric epithelium, and death. Chronic primary mycotoxicosis, resulting from moderate to low levels of mycotoxin intake, often cause reduced productivity in the form of slower rate of growth, reduced production and inferior market quality. Consumption of low levels of mycotoxins through the feeds do not cause serious mycotoxicosis, but often predisposes to various infectious diseases and especially to secondary bacterial infections [68, 69], because of the suppression in both humoral and cell mediated immune response in such animals [68].

6. Economic impacts of mycotoxins

Mycotoxins are estimated to affect as much as 25% of the world's crops each year [70]. In the United States and Canada alone, the cost of mycotoxins is estimated to be more than $5 billion each year [7]. In developing countries, many foods and feeds which otherwise can be available for consumption or trade are lost in production or storage [71]. The mycotoxins in animal feeds are one of the leading causes of output losses and increased management expenses in animal husbandry around the world [72].

Mycotoxin-contaminated products cause significant economic and trade problems at almost every marketing stage, from the producer to the consumer. Many importing countries have placed restrictions without following the Codex Alimentarius Commission's guidelines for risk assessment and acceptable methodologies thereby negatively impacting developing countries' economies [73]. Mycotoxins in ethanol co-products (dry distiller's grain and soluble) have an annual economic impact of about $18 million on the swine sector in the United States. Mycotoxins create economic losses because of their effects on cattle production, crop losses, and the costs of regulatory programs targeting mycotoxins. Depending on the toxicity of each mycotoxin and the country, regulation limits for mycotoxins in animal feedstuffs vary whereas in some countries the limits might not even exist [7, 74, 75].

Mycotoxins significantly impact both the productivity and the nutritional value of cereal and forage [70]. Molds use nutrients from the feed to grow. This results in reduced energy content of the feeds, decreased feed palatability and increased feed refusal by animals [64]. Consumption of feeds contaminated by mycotoxins cause organ damage, immune suppression and health disorders, limiting growth and performance of farm animals [76] and thereby directly leading to economic losses [77]. The economic impact of mycotoxins includes loss of animal and human life, increased health care and veterinary care costs, reduced livestock production, disposal of contaminated foods and feeds, and investment in research to reduce severity of the mycotoxin problem [78].

7. Risk management: prevention of mycotoxins in feeds

Because of the harmful consequences of these mycotoxins, several strategies have been developed to assist prevent the production of mycotoxigenic fungus, as well as detoxify mycotoxin-contaminated animal feeds. These includes:

- Mycotoxin contamination prevention.

- Mycotoxin detoxification in feed.
- Mycotoxin absorption inhibition in the gastrointestinal tract.

There are physical, chemical and biological treatment methods as well as commercially available products that can be added to the diet to reduce the harmful effects of mycotoxin-contaminated animal feed, in addition to pre- and postharvest prevention procedures to control mycotoxin contamination in feedstuffs and feed. Some of the new techniques for controlling mycotoxicosis in animals include enzymes, microbes, antibodies, aptamers, and transgenic crops although binders are the current widely used mycotoxin detoxifiers with varying results [7]. Therefore, to lessen the harmful and economic impact of mycotoxins in feeds, any detoxification technique must meet an essential criteria [63, 79]: The technique must either inactivate or remove the mycotoxins in feeds, avoid producing or leaving toxic residues, not alter the nutritional and technological properties of feed, be capable of destroying fungal spores to prevent the formation of new toxins, and be technically and economically feasible.

Contamination mainly occurs or is encouraged before harvest and during harvesting [80]. Currently researchers worldwide are keen on developing effective methods to prevent preharvest mycotoxin contamination. Preharvest preventive measures include breeding resistant crops, good agronomic practices such as irrigation to prevent plant stress and crop rotation to reduce soil population of mycotoxin producing fungi and harvesting at the optimum stage of maturity [81].

The control of insect infestation in kernels may help to prevent *A. flavus* and *A. parasiticus* proliferation and subsequent aflatoxin production [82]. The introduction of non-toxin producing isolates of *A. flavus* to competitively replace aflatoxin producers is one of the most promising strategies for reducing preharvest contamination of crops with aflatoxin [83]. A good quality product is obtained only when the crop is harvested at the optimum stage of maturity, particularly if it is to be stored subsequently for protracted periods [71]. İt is desirable to harvest early in the day, in the same cases, at the sunset to avoid excessive field heat leading to rapid deterioration and fungal colonization. Where harvesting is done in dry weather, mycotoxin contamination does not prove problematic, it does however pose a problem when harvesting is done in very humid weather [84]. Delayed harvest particularly favors contamination with *Fusarium*. Mechanically damaged and shriveled grains are regularly contaminated by molds, and moldy grains can partially be removed by separators [85].

Unless the moisture content is safe below the grain-moisture content, which is in equilibrium with humidity of the air component of the grain, the development of fungi and other spoilage organisms is almost inevitable. The easiest and cheapest way of ensuring safe storage is to reduce moisture content before storage. Thus, where natural reduction is prevented by natural conditions at harvest time, the grain must be dried before storage [65]. Mold problems only occur if silage is exposed to oxygen for instance if the silage is not tightly covered, in case of damaged covers or when silage is being fed out to the livestock. İt is recommended to use airtight containers during the ensiling process of forage and if these containers are damaged in any way, repairs must be made as quickly as possible to stop the development of mold [64].

While it is sensible to store feedstuffs under conditions of temperature and humidity that minimize fungal growth, it is often the case that the product has been spoiled before harvest and already contains a considerable amount of mycotoxins [86]. Thus, detoxification processes including biological, chemical and physical methods are often necessary to remove, destroy or reduce toxic effects, without producing or leaving toxic residues or carcinogens in the food and animal feed materials.

7.1 Physical strategies

Irradiation and thermal processing techniques like cooking, boiling, baking, frying, roasting, microwave heating, and extrusion are some of the physical techniques used for reducing or inactivating mycotoxins in feeds [45]. These physical methods including sorting, flotation, and extraction remove mycotoxins from contaminated grain products and/or eliminate the bioavailability of mycotoxins in the gastrointestinal system [87]. Heat treatments are applicable in degrading mycotoxins in feedstuffs. Of the toxins isolated from fungi, more than 90% melt at temperature above 100°C, and 70% have melting point above 150°C and 250°C. However, heat may destroy vitamins and denature proteins and so reduce nutritive value especially at the temperature required for degradation of mycotoxins [88].

7.2 Extraction with solvents

Mycotoxins can be extracted from contaminated food materials like oilseed peanuts and cottonseed using a variety of solvents. 95% ethanol, 90% aqueous acetone, aqueous isopropanol, 80% isopropanol, hexane-methanol, methanol-water, acetonitrile-water, hexane-ethanol-water, and acetone-hexane-water are the most often used solvents [84]. While solvent extraction can efficiently remove aflatoxin from oilseed meals without the creation of hazardous byproducts or a deterioration in nutritional properties, the technique's large-scale implementation is limited by its high cost and concerns with toxic extract disposal [84, 89].

7.3 Adsorption

One strategy for decreasing mycotoxin exposure is to reduce their bioavailability by incorporating various mycotoxin-adsorbing agents into the compound feed, which reduces mycotoxin uptake and transport to the blood and target organs. Adsorbing agents are substances of high molecular weight that, upon reaching the gastrointestinal system (aqueous medium), can bind mycotoxins, preventing their absorption, and allowing fecal excretion of this adsorbent–toxin complex [90]. They do not dissociate in the gastrointestinal tract of the animal thus preventing or minimizing exposure of animals to mycotoxins.

Mycotoxin-adsorbing agents can be silica-based inorganic compounds or carbon-based organic polymers. Some of the inorganic adsorbing agents utilized include natural clay products as well as synthetic polymers. Activated carbons, hydrated sodium calcium aluminosilicate (HSCAS), zeolites, bentonites, and certain clays are the most studied adsorbents, they possess a high affinity for mycotoxins, and they have shown immense potential for use in animal feeds to overcome aflatoxicosis [77, 84]. Adsorption agents are quite successful in preventing aflatoxicosis, although they are not as effective against other mycotoxins [91]. The main mycotoxins are adsorbed sufficiently by at least one type of adsorbent, but a few adsorbents may be used for various mycotoxins and none of them have been shown to be effective against all toxins (**Table 3**) [93].

When supplemented at a concentration of 10 g/kg feed, most of them have been shown to be effective aflatoxins binders. Their effectiveness against mycotoxins such as zearalenone, fumonisins, and trichothecenes, on the other hand, is very limited or

Compounds	Affected mycotoxins
Hydrated sodium calcium aluminosilicate (HSCAS)	Aflatoxin B1
Zeolites	Aflatoxin B1 and zearalenone
Bentonites	Aflatoxin B1 and T2 toxin
Specific clays (kaolin, sepiolite and montmorillonite)	Aflatoxin B1
Active carbons	Ochratoxin and aflatoxin B1
Colestiralamine	Ochratoxin and zearalenone
Poly-vinyl polypyrrolidone polymers (PVPP)	Aflatoxin B1

Table 3.
Some adsorbents and mycotoxins on which they are effective [92].

non-existent [77]. T-2 toxin can be adsorbed by bentonite, however its inclusion rate in the diet must be 10 times higher (100 g/kg) than the effective amount for aflatoxins [94]. Phyllosilicates such as kaolin and sepiolite, like most clays, are ineffective against mycotoxins other than aflatoxins [95, 96]. Because clay binders are relatively ineffective against mycotoxins other than aflatoxins, natural organic binders have been highly proposed. Organic binders are more effective against a wider spectrum of mycotoxins than inorganic binders, making them better suited to multi-contaminated diets. They're also biodegradable, which means they will not end up in the environment after being expelled by animals. Clays, on the other hand, which are assimilated at a faster pace than organics, collect in manure and then spread in the field, causing harm to the environment [96].

7.4 Chemical techniques

Mycotoxins have been found to be reduced, destroyed, or inactivated by a variety of chemicals. Acids (e.g., formic and propionic acids), bases (e.g., ammonia, sodium hydroxide), oxidizing compounds (e.g., hydrogen peroxide, ozone), reducing agents (e.g., bisulphite), chlorinating agents (e.g., sodium hypochlorite, chlorine dioxide, and gaseous chlorine), and miscellaneous reagents (e.g., formaldehyde) are some examples of these chemicals which have undergone testing before for their efficacy in mycotoxin decontamination [84, 85, 97]. Even though most of these chemical treatments can remove mycotoxins in feeds, chemical detoxification does not meet the FAO requirements, because they often reduce the nutrient quality of the treated feeds, and some compounds leave behind their toxic metabolites that have unfavorable side effects [84, 85]. This is the fundamental reason why their extensive use in the animal feeds sector is severely constrained.

7.5 Biological techniques

Biological detoxification implies the biotransformation or degradation of a toxin, by bio-transforming agents such as endogenous enzymes to a metabolite that is either non-toxic when ingested by animals or less toxic than the original toxin and readily excreted from the body. Because it works under mild, ecologically favorable circumstances, biological decomposition of mycotoxins has showed promise [98].

A variety of bacteria, yeasts, and molds can degrade aflatoxins. The idea is to utilize enzymes that precisely breakdown each mycotoxin, or class of mycotoxins, into a

	Mycotoxin	Binding capacity (%)
Lactobacillus rhamnosus species (G.G.)	Aflatoxin B1	80
Propionibacterium	Aflatoxin B1	80
Bifidobacterium bifidum species	Aflatoxin B2, G1, and G2	74, 80 and 80
Saccharomyces cerevisiae	Zearalenone	52
Glucomannan obtained from the cell wall	Aflatoxin	95
	Fumonisin	45
	Deoxynivalenol	10

Table 4.
The toxin binding capacity of biological products obtained from yeast cell walls with different bacterial species [92].

non-toxic molecule. With recent developments in molecular biology, genetic engineering, and microbial genomics, as well as the discovery of microbial populations' catabolic capacities, research in this area has expanded. It has been widely proven that microorganisms, such as fungus and bacteria, may breakdown mycotoxins in feed (**Table 4**) [99–101]. *Saccharomyces cerevisiae* is one of the most successful developing bacteria at binding to AFB1. Strains such as *Phoma* sp., *Mucor* sp., *Trichoderma harzianum*, *Trichoderma* sp. 639, *Rhizopus* sp. 663, *Rhizopus* sp. 710, *Rhizopus* sp. 668, *Alternaria* sp. and some strains belonging to the *Sporotrichum* group are some of the fungal strains that have been demonstrated to degrade AFB_1 to levels ranging from 65–99% [102].

Flavobacterium aurantiacum also shown the ability to effectively remove aflatoxin B1 [103]. Based on a European Food Safety survey, *Trichosporon mycotoxinivorans* was found to be the only microorganism that shows the potential to degrade OTA and meets the prerequisites for use as an animal feed additive [104]. Therefore, as endogenous oxidation control systems may be more desirable, extensive research is needed in identifying, characterizing and purifying enzymes involved before this approach becomes more practical [97, 103].

Enzyme-linked immunosorbent assays, thin layer chromatography, high performance liquid chromatography, gas chromatography, near-infrared spectroscopy, and liquid chromatography-mass spectrometry are some of the current analytical methods for detecting and quantifying mycotoxins. Some of these techniques can be applied to samples that contain numerous mycotoxins [7].

8. Conclusion

Mycotoxins are toxic secondary metabolites produced naturally by fungi that grow on various agricultural commodities. Mycotoxins significantly impact both the productivity and the nutritional value of cereal and forage. Mycotoxin contaminated feeds impact animal health and productivity. Contamination of feeds may occur during pre-harvest and post-harvest. Every year, mycotoxins cause massive economic losses in the animal feed sector and animal husbandry. As a result, measures to remove or inactivate mycotoxins in diet and feed are critical. Different measures to prevent mycotoxin production and its drawbacks are being applied worldwide. On farm measures are efficient in terms of products safety and costly feasible, but there are not enough to completely prevent fungi growth in crops. Therefore, detoxification

DOI: http://dx.doi.org/10.5772/intechopen.102010

processes including biological, chemical and physical methods are often used to remove, destroy or reduce toxic effects in feeds or food contaminated in the field. However, traditional physical and chemical procedures have several drawbacks, including limited efficacy, safety concerns, palatability losses, and the high cost of the equipment required to perform these techniques. They have also been criticized to reduce nutritive value of the feeds, and to have side effects on animal and human health. Adsorbents and microorganisms/enzymes use may be more desirable and are currently used as feed additives in many parts of the world. Further research work is needed to weigh out their potential compared to the other methods of detoxification.

Author details

Zacharia Waithaka Ng'ang'a[1,2*] and Eric Niyonshuti[2]

1 MoBioFood Research Group, Department of Biochemistry and Biotechnology, Universität Rovira i Virgili, Tarragona, Spain

2 Department of Animal Science, Ege University, Izmir, Turkey

*Address all correspondence to: zachariawaithaka96@gmail.com

IReferences

[1] FIF. Global Feed Statistics. International Feed Industry Federation; 2021. https://ifif.org/global-feed/statistics/ [Accessed: December 6, 2021]

[2] der Poel AFB van, Abdollahi MR, Cheng H, Colovic R, den Hartog LA, Miladinovic D, et al. Future directions of animal feed technology research to meet the challenges of a changing world. Animal Feed Science and Technology. 2020;**270**:114692. DOI: 10.1016/J.ANIFEEDSCI.2020.114692

[3] Pereira CS, Cunha SC, Fernandes JO. Prevalent mycotoxins in animal feed: Occurrence and analytical methods. Toxins. 2019;**11**:290. DOI: 10.3390/TOXINS11050290

[4] Edite Bezerra da Rocha M, Freire F d CO, Erlan Feitosa Maia F, Izabel Florindo Guedes M, Rondina D. Mycotoxins and their effects on human and animal health. Food Control. 2014;**36**:159-165. DOI: 10.1016/J.FOODCONT.2013.08.021

[5] Awuchi CG, Ondari EN, Ogbonna CU, Upadhyay AK, Baran K, Okpala COR, et al. Mycotoxins affecting animals, foods, humans, and plants: Types, occurrence, toxicities, action mechanisms, prevention, and detoxification strategies—a revisit. Food. 2021;**10**:1279. DOI: 10.3390/FOODS10061279

[6] Steyn PS. The biosynthesis of mycotoxins. Revue de Médecine Vétérinaire. 1998;**149**:469-478. DOI: 10.1016/B978-0-12-670650-5.X5001-8

[7] Madhysatha S, Marquardt RR. Mycotoxins in the feed and animal products. Poultry and Pig Nutrition. 2019:263-278. DOI: 10.3920/978-90-8686-884-1_12

[8] Chaytor AC, Hansen JA, van Heugten E, See MT, Kim SW. Occurrence and decontamination of mycotoxins in swine feed. Asian-Australasian Journal of Animal Sciences. 2011;**24**:723-738. DOI: 10.5713/AJAS.2011.10358

[9] Ismaiel AA, Papenbrock J. Mycotoxins: Producing fungi and mechanisms of phytotoxicity. Agriculture. 2015;**5**:492-537. DOI: 10.3390/AGRICULTURE5030492

[10] Galvano F, Ritieni A, Piva G, Pietri A. Mycotoxins in the Human Food Chain. In: Diaz DE, editor. The Mycotoxin Blue Book. Nottingham, UK: Nottingham University Press; 2005. p. 187-224

[11] D'mello JPF. Contaminants and toxins in animal feeds. In: Assessing Quality and Safety of Animal Feeds. Rome: Food and Agriculture Organization of the United Nations; 2004. pp. 107-128

[12] Santin E. Mould growth and mycotoxin production. In: Diaz DE, editor. The Mycotoxin Blue Book. Nottingham, UK: Nottingham University Press; 2005. pp. 225-234

[13] Gashaw M. Review on Mycotoxins in Feeds: Implications to Livestock and human health. E3 Journal of Agricultural Research and Development. 2015;**5**:137-0144

[14] CAST. Mycotoxins: Risks in Plant, Animal, and Human Systems. Ames, Iowa, USA: Agricultural Science and Technology; Agricultural Science and Technology; 2003

[15] Whitaker TB, Slate AB, Johansson AS. Sampling feeds for mycotoxin analysis. In: Diaz DE, editor. The Mycotoxin Blue

Book. Nottingham, UK: Nottingham University Press; 2005. pp. 1-23

[16] FAO. Worldwide Regulations for Mycotoxins 1995: A Compendium. Rome: Food and Agriculture Organization of the United Nations; 1997

[17] D'Mello JPF, Macdonald AMC. Mycotoxins. Animal Feed Science and Technology. 1997;**69**:155-166. DOI: 10.1016/S0377-8401(97)81630-6

[18] Moss MO. Environmental factors controlling mycotoxin formation. In: Smith D, Henderson R, editors. Mycotoxins and Animal Foods. CRC Press; 1991. p. 39

[19] Grenier B, Oswald IP. Mycotoxin co-contamination of food and feed: Meta-analysis of publications describing toxicological interactions. World Mycotoxin Journal. 2011;**4**:285-313. DOI: 10.3920/WMJ2011.1281

[20] Binder EM, Tan LM, Chin LJ, Handl J, Richard J. Worldwide occurrence of mycotoxins in commodities, feeds and feed ingredients. Animal Feed Science and Technology. 2007;**137**:265-282. DOI: 10.1016/j.anifeedsci.2007.06.005

[21] Cheeke PR, Shull LR. Natural Toxicants in Feeds and Poisonous Plants. Westport Conn: AVI Pub. Co; 1985

[22] Lillehoj EB, Cleveland TE, Bhatnagar D. Mycotoxins in feedstuffs: Production in novel substrates. In: Smith JE, Henderson RS, editors. Mycotoxins and Animal Foods. Boca Raton, FL, USA: CRC Press; 1991. pp. 399-413

[23] Alvarado AM, Zamora-Sanabria R, Granados-Chinchilla F. A focus on aflatoxins in feedstuffs: Levels of contamination, prevalence, control strategies, and impacts on animal health. In: Aflatoxin-Control, Analysis, Detection and Health Risks. London, UK: IntechOpen; 2017. pp. 115-152. DOI: 10.5772/INTECHOPEN.69468

[24] Elzupir AO, Younis YMH, Himmat Fadul M, Elhussein AM. Determination of aflatoxins in animal feed in Khartoum State, Sudan. Journal of Animal and Veterinary Advances. 2009;**8**:1000-1003

[25] Williams JG, Deschl U, Williams GM. DNA damage in fetal liver cells of turkey and chicken eggs dosed with aflatoxin B1. Archives of Toxicology. 2011;**85**:1167-1172. DOI: 10.1007/S00204-011-0653-X/FIGURES/3

[26] Gholami-Ahangaran M, Rangsaz N, Azizi S. Evaluation of turmeric (*Curcuma longa*) effect on biochemical and pathological parameters of liver and kidney in chicken aflatoxicosis. Pharmaceutical Biology. 2015;**54**:780-787. DOI: 10.3109/13880209.2015.1080731

[27] Sherazi STH, Shar ZH, Sumbal GA, Tan ET, Bhanger MI, Kara H, et al. Occurrence of ochratoxin A in poultry feeds and feed ingredients from Pakistan. Mycotoxin Research. 2015;**31**:1-7. DOI: 10.1007/S12550-014-0216-0/FIGURES/3

[28] Denli M, Perez JF. Ochratoxins in feed, a risk for animal and human health: Control strategies. Toxins. 2010;**2**:1065-1077. DOI: 10.3390/TOXINS2051065

[29] Reddy L, Bhoola K. Ochratoxins—Food contaminants: Impact on human health. Toxins. 2010;**2**:771-779. DOI: 10.3390/TOXINS2040771

[30] Heussner AH, Bingle LEH. COMPARATIVE ochratoxin toxicity: A review of the available data. Toxins. 2015;**7**:4253-4282. DOI: 10.3390/TOXINS7104253

[31] Malir F, Ostry V, Pfohl-Leszkowicz A, Novotna E, Ochratoxin A. Developmental

and reproductive toxicity—An overview. Birth Defects Research Part B: Developmental and Reproductive Toxicology. 2013;**98**:493-502. DOI: 10.1002/BDRB.21091

[32] Battacone G, Nudda A, Pulina G. Effects of ochratoxin A on livestock production. Toxins. 2010;**2**:1796-1824. DOI: 10.3390/TOXINS2071796

[33] Chang H, Kim W, Park JH, Kim D, Kim CR, Chung S, et al. The occurrence of zearalenone in South Korean feedstuffs between 2009 and 2016. Toxins. 2017;**9**:223. DOI: 10.3390/TOXINS9070223

[34] Maragos CM. Zearalenone occurrence and human exposure. World Mycotoxin Journal. 2010;**3**:369-383. DOI: 10.3920/WMJ2010.1240

[35] Gajęcki M. Zearalenone—undesirable substances in feed. Polish Journal of Veterinary Sciences. 2002;**5**:117-122

[36] Yumbe-Guevara BE, Imoto T, Yoshizawa T. Effects of heating procedures on deoxynivalenol, nivalenol and zearalenone levels in naturally contaminated barley and wheat. Food Additives & Contaminants. 2003;**20**:1132-1140. DOI: 10.1080/02652030310001620432

[37] Zinedine A, Soriano JM, Moltó JC, Mañes J. Review on the toxicity, occurrence, metabolism, detoxification, regulations and intake of zearalenone: An oestrogenic mycotoxin. Food and Chemical Toxicology. 2007;**45**:1-18. DOI 10.1016/J.FCT.2006.07.030

[38] Knutsen HK, Alexander J, Barregård L, Bignami M, Brüschweiler B, Ceccatelli S, et al. Risks for animal health related to the presence of zearalenone and its modified forms in feed. EFSA Journal. 2017;**15**:e04851. DOI: 10.2903/J.EFSA.2017.4851

[39] Fink-Gremmels J, Malekinejad H. Clinical effects and biochemical mechanisms associated with exposure to the mycoestrogen zearalenone. Animal Feed Science and Technology. 2007;**137**:326-341. DOI: 10.1016/J.ANIFEEDSCI.2007.06.008

[40] Stoev SD. Foodborne mycotoxicoses, risk assessment and underestimated hazard of masked mycotoxins and joint mycotoxin effects or interaction. Environmental Toxicology and Pharmacology. 2015;**39**:794-809. DOI: 10.1016/J.ETAP.2015.01.022

[41] Richard JL. Some major mycotoxins and their mycotoxicoses—An overview. International Journal of Food Microbiology. 2007;**119**:3-10. DOI: 10.1016/J.IJFOODMICRO.2007.07.019

[42] Gelderblom WCA, Marasas WFO, Jaskiewicz K, Combrinck S, van Schalkwyk DJ. Cancer promoting potential of different strains of *Fusarium moniliforme* in a short-term cancer initiation/promotion assay. Carcinogenesis. 1988;**9**:1405-1409. DOI: 10.1093/CARCIN/9.8.1405

[43] Hussein HS, Brasel JM. Toxicity, metabolism, and impact of mycotoxins on humans and animals. Toxicology. 2001;**167**:101-134. DOI: 10.1016/S0300-483X(01)00471-1

[44] Kovalsky P, Kos G, Nährer K, Schwab C, Jenkins T, Schatzmayr G, et al. Co-occurrence of regulated, masked and emerging mycotoxins and secondary metabolites in finished feed and maize—an extensive survey. Toxins. 2016;**8**:363. DOI: 10.3390/TOXINS8120363

[45] Aiko V, Mehta A. Occurrence, detection and detoxification of

mycotoxins. Journal of Biosciences. 2015;**40**:943-954. DOI: 10.1007/S12038-015-9569-6

[46] Mostrom M, Raisbeck MF. Trichothecenes. In: Ramesh C. Gupta, editor. Veterinary Toxicology. 2nd ed., Elsevier Inc; Academic Press; 2012. pp. 1239-1265. DOI: 10.1016/B978-0-12-385926-6.00108-3

[47] Wan Q, Wu G, He Q, Tang H, Wang Y. The toxicity of acute exposure to T-2 toxin evaluated by the metabonomics technique. Molecular BioSystems. 2015;**11**:882-891. DOI: 10.1039/C4MB00622D

[48] Awad W, Ghareeb K, Böhm J, Zentek J. The toxicological impacts of the fusarium mycotoxin, deoxynivalenol, in poultry flocks with special reference to immunotoxicity. Toxins. 2013;**5**:912-925. DOI: 10.3390/TOXINS5050912

[49] Prelusky DB, Hamilton RMG, Trenholm HL, Miller JD. Tissue distribution and excretion of radioactivity following administration of 14C-labeled deoxynivalenol to White Leghorn hens. Fundamental and Applied Toxicology. 1986;7:635-645. DOI: 10.1016/0272-0590(86)90113-2

[50] Hsu I-C, Smalley EB, Strong FM, Ribelin WE. Identification of T-2 toxin in moldy corn associated with a lethal toxicosis in dairy cattle. Applied Microbiology. 1972;**24**:684-690

[51] Marin S, Ramos AJ, Cano-Sancho G, Sanchis V. Mycotoxins: Occurrence, toxicology, and exposure assessment. Food and Chemical Toxicology. 2013;**60**:218-237. DOI: 10.1016/J.FCT.2013.07.047

[52] Jones FT, Genter MB, Hagler WM, Hansen JA, Mowrey BA, Poore MH, et al. Understanding and Coping with Effects of Mycotoxins in Livestock Feed and Forage Safe Levels of Mycotoxins. North Carolina: North Carolina Agricultural Extension Service, North Carolina University; 1994

[53] Akande KE, Abubakar MM, Adegbola TA, Bogoro SE. Nutritional and health implications of mycotoxins in animal feeds: A review. Pakistan Journal of Nutrition. 2006;**5**:398-403. DOI: 10.3923/PJN.2006.398.403

[54] Li Y, Wang Z, Beier RC, Shen J, Smet D de, de Saeger S, et al. T-2 toxin, a trichothecene mycotoxin: Review of toxicity, metabolism, and analytical methods. Journal of Agricultural and Food Chemistry 2011;59:3441-3453. DOI: 10.1021/JF200767Q

[55] Mishra S, Ansari KM, Dwivedi PD, Pandey HP, Das M. Occurrence of deoxynivalenol in cereals and exposure risk assessment in Indian population. Food Control. 2013;**30**:549-555. DOI: 10.1016/J.FOODCONT.2012.07.041

[56] Marasas WFO, Kriek NPJ, Fincham JE, van Rensburg SJ. Primary liver cancer and oesophageal basal cell hyperplasia in rats caused by *Fusarium moniliforme*. International Journal of Cancer. 1984;**34**:383-387. DOI: 10.1002/IJC.2910340315

[57] Chaytor AC, See MT, Hansen JA, de Souza ALP, Middleton TF, Kim SW. Effects of chronic exposure of diets with reduced concentrations of aflatoxin and deoxynivalenol on growth and immune status of pigs. Journal of Animal Science. 2011;**89**:124-135. DOI: 10.2527/JAS.2010-3005

[58] Wu L, Liao P, He L, Ren W, Yin J, Duan J, et al. Growth performance, serum biochemical profile, jejunal morphology, and the expression of nutrients transporter genes in deoxynivalenol (DON)-challenged growing pigs. BMC Veterinary

Research. 2015;**11**. DOI: 10.1186/S12917-015-0449-Y

[59] Maresca M. From the gut to the brain: Journey and pathophysiological effects of the food-associated trichothecene mycotoxin deoxynivalenol. Toxins. 2013;**5**:784-820. DOI: 10.3390/TOXINS5040784

[60] Hughes DM, Gahl MJ, Graham CH, Grieb SL. Overt signs of toxicity to dogs and cats of dietary deoxynivalenol. Journal of Animal Science. 1999;**77**: 693-700. DOI: 10.2527/1999.773693X

[61] Milani JM. Ecological conditions affecting mycotoxin production in cereals: A review. Veterinarni Medicina. 2018;**58**:405-411. DOI: 10.17221/6979-VETMED

[62] Jarvis B. Factors affecting the production of mycotoxins. Journal of Applied Bacteriology. 1971;**34**:199-213. DOI: 10.1111/J.1365-2672.1971.TB02278.X

[63] Zaki MM, El-Midany SA, Shaheen HM, Rizzi L. Mycotoxins in animals: Occurrence, effects, prevention and management. Journal of Toxicology and Environmental Health Sciences. 2012;**4**:13-28. DOI: 10.5897/JTEHS11.072

[64] Golob P. On-farm mycotoxin control in food and feed grain. In: Good Practices for Animal Feed and Livestock Training Manual. Rome, Italy: FAO; 2007. p. 27

[65] Williams PC. Storage of grains and seeds. In: Smith JE, Henderson RS, editors. Mycotoxins and Animal Foods. Boca Raton, FL: CRC Press; 1991. p. 738

[66] Morgavi DP, Riley RT. An historical overview of field disease outbreaks known or suspected to be caused by consumption of feeds contaminated with Fusarium toxins. Animal Feed Science and Technology. 2007;**137**:201-212. DOI: 10.1016/J.ANIFEEDSCI.2007.06.002

[67] Kan CA, Meijer GAL. The risk of contamination of food with toxic substances present in animal feed. Animal Feed Science and Technology. 2007;**133**:84-108. DOI: 10.1016/j.anifeedsci.2006.08.005

[68] Stoev SD, Anguelov G, Ivanov I, Pavlov D. Influence of ochratoxin A and an extract of artichoke on the vaccinal immunity and health in broiler chicks. Experimental and Toxicologic Pathology. 2000;**52**:43-55. DOI: 10.1016/S0940-2993(00)80014-7

[69] Koynarski V, Stoev S, Grozeva N, Mirtcheva T, Daskalov H, Mitev J, et al. Experimental coccidiosis provoked by *Eimeria acervulina* in chicks simultaneously fed on ochratoxin A contaminated diet. Research in Veterinary Science. 2007;**82**:225-231. DOI: 10.1016/J.RVSC.2006.07.004

[70] Iheshiulor OOM, Esonu BO, Chuwuka OK, Omede AA, Okoli IC, Ogbuewu IP. Effects of mycotoxins in animal nutrition: A review. Asian Journal of Animal Sciences. 2011;**5**:19-33. DOI: 10.3923/AJAS.2011.19.33

[71] Aidoo KE. Storage and preservation of tropical crops. In: Smith JE, Henderson RS, editors. Mycotoxins and Animal Foods. Boca Raton, FL: CRC Press; 1991. pp. 747-764

[72] Adamse P, Egmond HJ van, Driessen JJM, de Rijk TC, de Jong J, de Nijs WCM. Trend Analysis of Mycotoxins in Animal Feed. Wageningen: Rikilt-Institute for Food Safety; 2012. (Rikilt report; 2011.017)

[73] Baht RV, Vashanti S. Occurrence of aflatoxin and its economic impact on human nutrition and animal feed: the new regulations. Cirad–Agritrop, Agriculture et Développement. 1999;23: 54-55. Available from: https://agritrop.cirad.fr/476183/

[74] Charmley LL, Trenholm HL. RG-8 regulatory guidance: Contaminants in feed. Section 1: Mycotoxins in livestock feed. In: Fact Sheet-Mycotoxins. Canada: Canadian Food Inspection Agency; 2012

[75] Streit E, Schatzmayr G, Tassis P, Tzika E, Marin D, Taranu I, et al. Current situation of mycotoxin contamination and co-occurrence in animal feed—focus on Europe. Toxins. 2012;**4**:788-809. DOI: 10.3390/TOXINS4100788

[76] Nadziakiewicza M, Kehoe S, Micek P. Physico-chemical properties of clay minerals and their use as a health promoting feed additive. Animals. 2019;**9**:714. DOI: 10.3390/ANI9100714

[77] Huwig A, Freimund S, Käppeli O, Dutler H. Mycotoxin detoxication of animal feed by different adsorbents. Toxicology Letters. 2001;**122**:179-188. DOI: 10.1016/S0378-4274(01)00360-5

[78] Zain ME. Impact of mycotoxins on humans and animals. Journal of Saudi Chemical Society. 2011;**15**:129-144. DOI: 10.1016/J.JSCS.2010.06.006

[79] Jemmali M. Decontamination and detoxification of mycotoxins. Pure and Applied Chemistry. 1980;**52**:175-181. DOI: 10.1351/PAC198052010175

[80] Omotayo OP, Omotayo AO, Mwanza M, Babalola OO. Prevalence of mycotoxins and their consequences on human health. Toxicological Research. 2019;**35**:1-7. DOI: 10.5487/TR.2019.35.1.001

[81] Xu F, Baker RC, Whitaker TB, Luo H, Zhao Y, Stevenson A, et al. Review of good agricultural practices for smallholder maize farmers to minimise aflatoxin contamination. World Mycotoxin Journal. 2021:1-16. DOI: 10.3920/WMJ2021.2685

[82] Lopez-garcia R, Park D, Phillips T. Integrated mycotoxin management systems. Food, Nutrition and Agriculture. 1999:38-48

[83] Moral J, Garcia-Lopez MT, Camiletti BX, Jaime R, Michailides TJ, Bandyopadhyay R, et al. Present status and perspective on the future use of aflatoxin biocontrol products. Agronomy. 2020;**10**:491. DOI: 10.3390/agronomy 10040491

[84] Kabak B, Dobson ADW, Var I. Strategies to prevent mycotoxin contamination of food and animal feed: A review. Critical Reviews in Food Science and Nutrition. 2007;**46**:593-619. DOI: 10.1080/10408390500436185

[85] Peraica M, Domijan A-M, Jurjević Ž, Cvjetković B. Prevention of exposure to mycotoxins from food and feed. Arhiv za Higijenu Rada i Toksikologiju. 2002;**53**:229-237

[86] Pemberton A, Simpson T. The chemical degradation of mycotoxins. In: Smith J, Henderson R, editors. Mycotoxins and Animal Feeding Stuffs: Natural Occurrence, Toxicity and Control. CRC Press; 1991. pp. 797-813

[87] He J, Zhou T. Patented techniques for detoxification of mycotoxins in feeds and food matrices. Recent Patents on Food, Nutrition & Agriculturee. 2010;**2**:96-104. DOI: 10.2174/2212798411002020096

[88] Samarajeewa U. In situ degradation of mycotoxins by physical methods. In: Smith J, Henderson R, editors. Mycotoxins and Animal Foods. Boca Raton, USA: CRC Press; 1991. pp. 785-796

[89] Rustom IYS. Aflatoxin in food and feed: Occurrence, legislation and inactivation by physical methods. Food Chemistry. 1997;**59**:57-67. DOI: 10.1016/S0308-8146(96)00096-9

[90] Santos GA, Rodrigues I, Starkl V, Naehrer K, Hofstetter U, Encarnação P. Mycotoxins in aquaculture: Occurrence in feeds components and impact on animal performance. Avances En Nutrición Acuicola. 2010:502-513

[91] Stoev SD. Food Safety and Increasing Hazard of Mycotoxin Occurrence in Foods and Feeds. Critical Reviews in Food Science and Nutrition. 2013;**53**:887-901. DOI: 10.1080/10408398.2011.571800

[92] Basmacıoğlu H, Ergül M, Üniversitesi E, Fak Z, Bölümü Z, Ve Y, et al. Yemlerde Bulunan Toksinler ve Kontrol Yolları. Hayvansal Üretim. 2003;**44**:9-17

[93] Di Gregorio MC, Neeff DV De, Jager AV, Corassin CH, Carão ÁCDP, Albuquerque R De, et al. Mineral adsorbents for prevention of mycotoxins in animal feeds. Toxin Reviews 2014;33:125-135. DOI: 10.3109/15569543.2014.905604

[94] Carson MS, Smith TK. Role of bentonite in prevention of T-2 toxicosis in rats. Journal of Animal Science. 1983;**57**:1498-1506. DOI: 10.2527/JAS1983.5761498X

[95] Schell TC, Lindemann MD, Kornegay ET, Blodgett DJ, Doerr JA. Effectiveness of different types of clay for reducing the detrimental effects of aflatoxin-contaminated diets on performance and serum profiles of weanling pigs. Journal of Animal Science. 1993;**71**:1226-1231. DOI: 10.2527/1993.7151226X

[96] Jouany JP. Methods for preventing, decontaminating and minimizing the toxicity of mycotoxins in feeds. Animal Feed Science and Technology. 2007;**137**:342-362. DOI: 10.1016/J.ANIFEEDSCI.2007.06.009

[97] Abdel-Wahh MA, Kholif AM. Mycotoxins in animal feeds and prevention strategies: A review. Asian Journal of Animal Sciences. 2008;**2**:7-25. DOI: 10.3923/AJAS.2008.7.25

[98] Ji C, Fan Y, Zhao L. Review on biological degradation of mycotoxins. Animal Nutrition. 2016;**2**:127-133. DOI: 10.1016/J.ANINU.2016.07.003

[99] Xia X, Zhang Y, Li M, Garba B, Zhang Q, Wang Y, et al. Isolation and characterization of a *Bacillus subtilis* strain with aflatoxin B1 biodegradation capability. Food Control. 2017;**75**:92-98. DOI: 10.1016/J.FOODCONT.2016.12.036

[100] Kabak B, Var I. Factors affecting the removal of aflatoxin M1 from food model by Lactobacillus and Bifidobacterium strains. Journal of Environmental Science and Health, Part B. 2008;**43**:617-624. DOI: 10.1080/03601230802234740

[101] Gerbaldo GA, Barberis C, Pascual L, Dalcero A, Barberis L. Antifungal activity of two Lactobacillus strains with potential probiotic properties. FEMS Microbiology Letters. 2012;**332**:27-33. DOI: 10.1111/J.1574-6968.2012.02570.X

[102] Shantha T. Fungal degradation of aflatoxin B1. Natural Toxins. 1999;7:175-178

[103] Bhatnagar D, Lillehoj EB, Bennet JW. Biological detoxification of mycotoxins. In: Smith JE, Henderson RS, editors. Mycotoxin and Animal Feeds. Boston: CRC Press; 1991. pp. 816-826

[104] Varga J, Kocinfé S, Péteri Z, Vágvölgyi C, Tóth B. Chemical, physical and biological approaches to prevent ochratoxin induced toxicoses in humans and animals. Toxins. 2010;**2**:1718-1750. DOI: 10.3390/TOXINS2071718

Section 4

Indirect Mycotoxin Contamination of Food Safety

Chapter 5

Food Safety Endangers the Potential *Escherichia coli* Contamination on Currencies

Dewi Susanna, Tris Eryando, Budi Hartono and Lassie Fitria

Abstract

Hands have a role in the transmission of pathogen of microbes such as virus, fungi, and bacteria. The transmission is often through the contact between hands and mouth. When money touches with sundries, there is a possibility of transfer of micro-organisms from hands to money and vice versa, then the dirty money will be held by someone else. Contamination of money is vital for public health problems because it can be a source of easy transmission of pathogens between handlers. Literacy related to how important is the *Escherichia coli* transmission through currencies is needed and also the way to measure its contamination. This paper describes the possibilities the existence of *E. coli* found on the surface of two types of currencies for instance papers and coins, and the steps to measure the contamination are also given in the Methods section.

Keywords: *Escherichia coli*, coin, currency, food safety, paper, transmission

1. Introduction

Escherichia coli (*E. coli*) is commonly found in the intestines of humans and warm-blooded animals, and most of the strains of *E. coli* are harmless. Shiga toxin-producing *E. coli* (STEC) can cause severe foodborne illness. It is transmitted to humans primarily through consuming contaminated food, such as raw or under-cooked ground meaty products, raw milk, and contaminated raw vegetables and sprouts [1]. Person-to-person transmission has been partially identified as a source of the pathogen. Hands have a role in the transmission of bacteria. People often touch objects already held by others and often put their hands to their mouths [2]. Besides that, *E. coli* can be moved from one object to the other with the help of human hands. One of the objects most often contaminated with *E. coli* is money. Money is a means of economic transactions that quickly move from one person to another. When money touches with sundries, there is a possibility of transfer of microorganisms from around to money. Then the dirty money will be held by someone else and so on. Contamination of money is vital for public health because it can be a means of easy transmission of pathogens between handlers.

Both coins and banknotes are frequently identified as materials for various microorganisms [3]. Fomites are inanimate objects capable of absorbing, storing, and transmitting infectious microorganisms [4]. Whether in the form of coins or banknotes, money is probably the item most people handle daily worldwide. It may become contaminated with microorganisms from the respiratory and gastrointestinal tracts during counting using saliva, coughing and sneezing on hands followed by currency exchange, placement or storage on dirty surfaces, poor handwashing after toilet. The banknote then acts as a bacterial vehicle to the following user [5, 6]. Most pathogens such as *Escherichia coli* can survive on surfaces, and this surface can act as a source of pathogen transmission if no disinfection is carried out. In addition, the level of general hygiene of a community or society can contribute to the number of microbes found on coins and banknotes, and thus the possibility of transmission during the handling of money.

Currency notes could potentially function as a fomite in transmitting microorganisms such as *E. coli* O157:H7 that cause enteric disease in humans. *Escherichia coli* is one of the microorganisms often found on the surface of an object, including the surface of the money. The research done in one of the meat markets in Nigeria showed that of the 189 samples, 12 (19.7%) were contaminated with *E. coli*, where (41.7%) are confirmed *E. coli* O157:H7 [7].

Another study showed that banknotes assessed through microbiological culture, microscopic visualization, and biochemical techniques identified *E. coli* contamination of about 4.75% [8]. While the currency used by the public (banks, hospitals, municipal corporation) in India was found to be highly contaminated with various pathogenic bacteria [9]. In Bangladesh, among banknotes, it was contaminated with three different bacterial isolates, including *E. coli* (87.5%). They were resistant to amoxicillin, ampicillin, and ciprofloxacin, susceptible to azithromycin and norfloxacin [10].

In Indonesia, it is quite difficult to find literacy that identifies *E. coli* on the surface of money. A study conducted in 2007 showed that there was *E. coli* on the surface of a 1000-rupiah bill in a community trader at Pasar Kleco, Surakarta [11].

2. The existence of *Escherichia coli* on currencies

2.1 Papers

The presence of bacteria on banknotes is strongly influenced by the material made of banknotes [3]. Banknotes are made from fibers that are coarse and provide an environment that is comfortable for the bacteria to survive. In addition, bacteria will have more surviving life in money paper that made fibers naturally dissolve in the mixed material plastic. Money paper does not give effect toxic on bacteria.

Research on Iranian currency also shows that *Escherichia coli* is the microorganism with the highest percentage in each type of currency [12]. This study also proves that the physical condition of money also affects the number of microorganisms on its surface. The more soiled the condition, the greater the number of microorganisms on its surface.

Research conducted by Gedik in 2013 concluded that the material that forms and composes money significantly affects the presence of microorganisms on the surface of money [13]. Banknote paper is manufactured from cotton fiber, which gives the paper its strength, durability, and distinctive feel. The cotton is sometimes mixed with linen, abaca, or other textile fibers. Banknote paper is infused with polyvinyl alcohol or gelatin to give it extra strength. This study also proves that Romanian banknotes are currencies whose ingredients can support the survival of microorganisms. In the same study, a microorganism transfer test was carried out on three respondents; the results showed that three respondents holding Romanian money were contaminated by the same microorganism [13]. The results of this study can be considered for countries that use money with the same materials and ingredients, especially for countries whose currencies are used globally, such as the US dollar and the euro.

Susanna, in 2019, researched banknotes and coins circulating at one of the universities in Depok, Indonesia. The communities taken are students and traders in the canteen. The sample money is money with large values such as 50,000 rupiahs to low-value banknotes, namely 1000 rupiahs. Based on the laboratory analysis results, there were no *E. coli* on the surface of the money, but there was still money contaminated with coliform [14]. This condition may occur because most money circulating is in good condition. The money holders have good knowledge regarding cleanliness because they are in an educational environment, so that the habit of washing hands can become one of the habits often done. The University of Indonesia already has a healthy canteen program under university management, which has provided education regarding personal hygiene to traders in the canteen.

2.2 Coins

Escherichia coli can survive on some metal surfaces, and *E. coli* O157 can survive for over 28 days at refrigeration and room temperatures on stainless steel [15]. Studies of *E. coli* on coins are not as much as studies on banknotes; this may be because the number of banknotes in circulation is far more than coins. Money and meager value denomination coins change hands frequently in poorer societies, unlike the people using plastic money. Generally, knowledge regarding personal hygiene in poorer societies is minimal, so this is an excellent factor contributing to the presence of microorganisms on coins. A study conducted by Curia in 2009 took samples of coins from contractor workers, food traders, and meat traders. The results showed that there were bacteria such as *E. coli* and fungi on the surface of the coins [4].

The presence of bacteria on coins does not last as long as on banknotes due to the direct toxic effect of coins on bacteria [3]. However, bacteria can adapt to the presence of coinage in their environment and increase their life span by the time they have adapted to the presence of coinage.

Like paper money, Susanna in 2019 also researched coins circulating at one of the universities in Depok, Indonesia. The sample money is money worth 1000 Indonesia Rupiah (IDR) to 100 IDR. Based on the laboratory analysis results, there were no *E. coli* on the surface of the money, but there was still money contaminated with coliform [14].

3. *Escherichia coli* detection on currencies

3.1 Materials and methods

The method used is total plate count (TPC) [7]. The working principle of TPC analysis is the calculation of the number of bacterial colonies present in the sample by dilution as needed and carried out in duplicate. All work is carried out aseptically to prevent unwanted contamination, and multiple observations can improve accuracy. The number of bacterial colonies that can be counted is a petri dish that has bacterial colonies between 30 and 300 colonies [16].

3.2 Isolation and identification of *E. coli*

There are several media used to isolate microorganisms in agar, including potato dextrose agar (PDA) [17], mannitol salt agar (MSA), xylose lysine deoxycholate (XLD) agar, MacConkey agar (MAC), eosin methylene blue (EMB) agar, bile salts citrate thiosulfate (TCBS) agar, *Bacillus cereus* (BCAM) agar base media [7]. Holt-Harris and Teague developed EMB agar (eosin methylene blue agar) media in 1916. EMB agar medium is selective for growing Gram-negative bacteria. They are generally used to separate and distinguish non-fecal coliform and fecal coliform bacteria. EMB can distinguish between bacterial colonies that can ferment lactose and those that cannot ferment the lactose [18, 19]. EMB agar consists of peptic digest of animal tissue 10,000 (GMS/L), dipotassium phosphate 2000 (GMS/L), lactose 5000 (GMS/L), sucrose 5000 (GMS/L), eosin-Y 0.400 (GMS/L), methylene blue 0.065 agar 13.500 (GMS/L), final pH (at 25°C) 7.2 ± 0.2 [18].

3.3 Total eligible count

The total viable count (TVC) is a simple way to dissect the microbial community's composition. It is used to indicate the different types and numbers of bacteria in a given sample. It is possible to isolate various bacteria from a single environmental sample, whether a soil sample or a wound swab [20].

Total feasible amount serial dilutions were made from 1 mL sample and 9 mL standard saline solution, two drops surface plated on plate count agar (PCA) for TVC. Plates were incubated at 37°C for 24 h. The number of different colonies on each plate was calculated using a colony counter, colony-forming units (CFU) per mL or cm^2 of the sample were calculated using the respective dilution factors and converted to log10, CFU/cm, or mL values.

4. Conclusion

Whether in the form of paper or coins, money is one of the media that can be a source of *E. coli* contamination. *Escherichia coli* has a reasonably long life on the surface of money, especially on coins that provide comfortable conditions for *E. coli* to survive, such as rough surfaces, natural fiber materials, and room temperature.

The existence of *E. coli* in money is very dependent on the cleanliness of the person holding the money (handler) when a money holder who has activities at risk of being contaminated with *E. coli*, such as food vendors and butchers, does not have the habit of washing hands, *E. coli* will quickly pass from hand to hand into someone else's hands.

Acknowledgements

The authors are grateful to the Ministry of Research and Technology of the Republic of Indonesia for granting financial support in contract no. NKB-47/UN2. RST/HKP.05.00/2020.

Conflict of interest

The authors declare no conflict of interest.

Author details

Dewi Susanna[1]*, Tris Eryando[2], Budi Hartono[1] and Lassie Fitria[3]

1 Department of Environmental Health, Faculty of Public Health, Universitas Indonesia, Indonesia

2 Department of Biostatistics and Population Studies, Faculty of Public Health, Universitas Indonesia, Indonesia

3 Master Program in Public Health, Faculty of Public Health, Universitas Indonesia, Indonesia

*Address all correspondence to: dsusanna@ui.ac.id; dsusanna2@yahoo.com

References

[1] World Health Organization (WHO). *E. coli* [Internet]. 2019. Available from: https://www.who.int/news-room/fact-sheets/detail/e-coli

[2] Jiang X, Doyle MP. Fate of *Escherichia coli* O157:H7 and *Salmonella enteritidis* on currency. Journal of Food Protection. 1999;**62**(7):805-807

[3] Vriesekoop F, Chen J, Oldaker J, Besnard F, Smith R, Leversha W, et al. Dirty money: A matter of bacterial survival, adherence, and toxicity. Microorganisms. 2016;**4**(4):42. Available from: http://www.mdpi.com/2076-2607/4/4/42 [Accessed: December 27, 2019]

[4] Angelakis E, Azhar EI, Bibi F, Yasir M, Al-Ghamdi AK, Ashshi AM, et al. Paper money and coins as potential vectors of transmissible disease. Future Microbiology. 2014;**9**(2):249-261

[5] Igumbor EO, Obi CL, Bessong PO, Potgieter N, Mkasi TC. Microbiological analysis of banknotes circulating in the Venda region of Limpopo province, South Africa. South African Journal of Science. 2007;**103**(9-10):365-366

[6] Hiko A, Abdata K, Muktar Y, Woyesa M, Mohammed A. Contamination of Ethiopian paper currency notes from various food handlers with *E. coli*. SpringerPlus. 2016;**5**(1):1065

[7] Mbaya PY, Junaidu AU, Raji MA, Ieren II. Evaluation of occurrence of *Escherichia coli* O157:H7 from Nigerian currency notes (Naira) collected from Butchers at the meat market in Karu Abattoir, Nigeria. IOSR Journal of Agriculture and Veterinary Science. 2016;**9**(12):34-39

[8] Muqtader Ahmed M, Fatima F, Javed Ansari M, Al-Shdefat R, Khalid Anwer M, Jamil S, et al. Bacterial contamination of Saudi Arabian paper currency: A report from Al-Kharj. Advancements in Life Sciences Journal. 2017;**4**(2):27-32

[9] Kalaskar A, Krishnappa K. A study of bacterial contamination of Indian currency notes in circulation. Indian Journal of Public Health Research and Development. 2014;**5**(2):295-299

[10] Barua N, Al A, Sabuj M, Haque ZF, Das M. Survey of bacterial contamination and antibiotic resistance pattern of Bangladeshi paper currency notes in Mymensingh city. African Journal of Microbiology Research. 2019;**13**(10):206-213

[11] Falah A. Deteksi Bakteri *Escherichia coli* Pada Uang Kertas Seribu yang beredar di Masyarakat [Internet]. Muhammadiyah Surakarta; 2007. Available from: http://eprints.ums.ac.id/10902/

[12] Moosavy MH, Shavisi N, Warriner K, Mosta-Favi E. Bacterial contamination of Iranian paper currency. Iranian Journal of Public Health. 2013;**42**(9):1067-1070

[13] Gedik H, Voss TA, Voss A. Money and transmission of bacteria. Antimicrobial Resistance and Infection Control. 2013;**2**(1):1

[14] Susanna D, Eryando T, Hartono B. Potensi Cemaran *Escherichia coli* di sekitar lingkungan Universitas Indonesia. Depok; 2019.

[15] Wilks SA, Michels H, Keevil CW. The survival of *Escherichia coli* O157 on a range of metal surfaces. International

Journal of Food Microbiology. 2005;**105**(3):445-454

[16] Mailoa MN, Tapotubun AM, Matrutty Theodora EAA. Analysis total plate counte (TPC) on fresh steak tuna applications edible coating Caulerpa sp. during stored at chilling temperature. In: IOP Conference Series: Earth and Environmental Science PAPER. Maluku, Indonesia: IOP Publishing Ltd; 2017. pp. 0-6

[17] Sadawarte K, Mahobe H, Saxena G. Microbial contamination of Indian currency notes in Bhopal. Journal of Evolution of Medical and Dental Sciences. 2014;**3**(6):1379-1384

[18] Lal A, Cheeptham N. Eosin-Methylene Blue Agar Plates Protocol. ASM Microbe Libr [Internet]. 2007. pp. 1-7. Available from: http://www.microbelibrary.org/component/resource/laboratory-test/2869-eosin-methylene-blue-agar-plates-protocol

[19] Holt-Haris J, Teague O. A new culture medium for the isolation of *Bacillus typhous* from stools. Journal of Infectious Diseases. 1915;**18**(6):596-600

[20] Total Viable Count—an overview|ScienceDirect Topics [Internet]. Available from: https://www.sciencedirect.com/topics/immunology-and-microbiology/total-viable-count [Accessed: December 28, 2019]

Section 5

Control and Reduction of Mycotoxin Contamination

Chapter 6

Cunninghamella bertholletiae's Toxins from Decomposing Cassava: Mitigation Strategy for Toxin Reduction Using *Nepenthes mirabilis* 'Monkey Cup' Digestive Fluids

Elie Fereche Itoba-Tombo, Seteno Karabo Obed Ntwampe, John Baptist Nzukizi Mudumbi, Lukhanyo Mekuto, Enoch Akinbiyi Akinpelu and Nkosikho Dlangamandla

Abstract

A fermentation technique was utilised to assess a fungus, i.e. *Cunninghamella bertholletiae/polymorpha*, isolated from rotting cassava, ability to produce mycotoxins and resultant oxidation by-products of the mycotoxins using liquid chromatography–mass spectrometry (LC/MS). Thus, the mycotoxins/secondary metabolites, fumonisin B^1 (FB^1) and deoxynivalenol (DON) were produced while, heptadecanone, octadecanamide, octadecenal and 3-keto-deoxynivalenol (DON) were successfully identified as biodegradation by-products in the fermentation broth treated with hydrolysing 'monkey cup' juice from *Nepenthes mirabilis*. Exposure to the mycotoxins and the biodegradation by-products through consumption of contaminated produce including contact due to the cumulative presence in arable agricultural soil can be harmful to humans and animals. Therefore, this work reports on a strategy for the mitigation and reduction of mycotoxins in agricultural soil using natural plant pitcher juices from *N. mirabilis*' 'monkey cup'.

Keywords: biodegradation, carboxylesterases, *Cunninghamella bertholethiae*, LC/MS, mycotoxins, *Nepenthes mirabilis*

1. Introduction

Postharvest storage for cassava is often shortened due to product spoilage caused by bacterial and fungal infestation [1, 2]. Fungal species such as *Aspergillus* spp., *Fusarium* spp., *Penicillium* spp. and *Cunninghamella* spp. can produce toxins and/or secondary metabolites that affect the storage longevity and quality of agricultural product such as cassava [2, 3]. These mycotoxins, which have a negative impact on agricultural products, lead to economic losses due to the contamination of cassava tubers, which makes them inedible. Generally, toxins are biosynthetic compounds produced by numerous microorganisms in a natural or controlled environment.

These microorganisms include the fungus, *Cunninghamella bertholletiae* (also known as *Cunninghamella polymorpha* due to its morphological characteristics and mating/reproductive scheme) [4], is known to be pathogenic to humans and animals [5–7], while its toxins in the environment and on consumable commodities constitute an environmental hazard and a health risk to consumers [8–11]. Some fungi, including their metabolites, are able to contaminate several plant parts as they are endophytes, culminating in infestation of agricultural products such as tomatoes, maize, potatoes, beans, peanuts, yams and wheat, including cassava [1, 5, 12–17] and dairy products such as milk and cheese [1, 18, 19]. Humans' or animals' consumption of contaminated products may lead to foodborne toxin-related intoxication [7, 20] culminating in the degeneration of human internal organs including their functionality and the promotion of diseases such as cancer [8, 15, 21–23]. Some clinical outcomes in animals and humans include liver and oesophageal cancer [21, 23], the destruction of renal and nerve tissues, profound oxidative stress, heart and pulmonary diseases [23].

There are several varieties of mycotoxins, namely aflatoxins (AFB^1, AFB^2, AFG^1 and AFG^2), fumonisins (FB^1, FB^2), deoxynivalenol (DON), ochratoxins (A, B and C), amongst others, which are produced by numerous species, some of which are deleterious to plants/agricultural products, humans and animals [1, 5, 21, 23, 24]. Their production can occur under favourable environmental conditions, such as a high temperature and adequate moisture/humidity, including the availability of nutrients (mostly from the decaying produce) [25]. These concerns have prompted researchers to find cheap, efficient and cost-effective ways to reduce or manage mycotoxin-producing organisms, including mycotoxin contamination, when produced [11, 26] to limit sequential effects including products' contamination.

In a previous study, it was found that *C. bertholletiae/polymorpha*, a common soil organism [7, 23, 26] which was isolated from decomposing cassava, was both cyanide-resistant with the ability to biodegrade free cyanide while being antagonistic towards other soil organisms [15, 27]. Currently, there is minimal literature available on mycotoxins produced by *C. bertholletiae*. Similarly, there is minimal research on a mitigation strategy which could be classified as environmentally benign for combined toxin reduction, via oxidation or hydrolysis. The mitigation method must be implementable *in-situ* in order to minimise deleterious effects observed when other methods are used.

Therefore, the aim of this study was to propose and assess a method for the identification of mycotoxins from the free-cyanide tolerant *C. bertholletiae/polymorpha* isolate; furthermore, to quantitatively assess a mitigation method using oxidative/hydrolysing 'monkey cup' digestive fluids from *N. mirabilis* (green chemistry approach). A *N. mirabilis* is a carnivorous plant which belongs to the genus of *Nepenthes*. This plant is characterised by a pitfall trap commonly known as a 'monkey cup' at the end of the plants' leaf, which contains an acidic and oxidative/hydrolysing fluid. The plants' pitcher juices are known to contain a variety of enzymes useful for prey digestion [28, 29]. As such, these enzymes can oxidise and/or hydrolyse mycotoxins and secondary metabolites via deamination or mechanisms biocatalytically facilitated by esterases for the decoupling of aliphatic chains in mycotoxins or secondary metabolites.

2. Mycotoxin (secondary metabolite) production in food

Several studies discussed about the presence of mycotoxins in food. Thus, during a produce life cycle from harvest, postharvest, selves' life, processing and sometimes distribution, there is a presence of mycotoxins in food worldwide [1]. These toxins occurred during poor storage, handling and processing conditions, sometimes might be the result of the rot/decay foodstuffs [2, 14, 30]. While these mycotoxins constitute a serious threat to food quality and human's health [22, 30].

2.1 Extraction and analysis of mycotoxins (secondary metabolites) and their biodegradation by-products

Literatures abound on the extraction and analysis of mycotoxins, a liquid-phase extraction method seems to be more used. Thus, [31, 32] used liquid-liquid extraction method for their studies in mycotoxins identification, while [33] used a liquid chromatography/tandem mass spectrometry for a combined analysis of aflatoxins, ochratoxin A and *Fusarium* for maize crop. Whereas [34] chose a multiplex approach of Gas chromatography–mass spectrometry (GC-MS), Liquid chromatography-mass spectrometry (LC-MS) and One-dimensional (1D) NMR spectroscopy (1D NMR) techniques for their study on a comparative metabolite profiling and fingerprinting of medicinal licorice roots, to name few.

The samples were analysed using an LC/MS-ToF 6230 (Agilent Technologies Inc., USA) and using mobile-phase parameters as listed in the table below in Supplementary Material, without optimisation as suggested by [31, 34]. The solvent extract phase was steadily evaporated using a blow-down technique to dryness at an ambient temperature for 24 h to minimise mycotoxin evaporation using nitrogen (N2) gas (Afrox, South Africa) [31, 35].

The identification of the mycotoxins from *C. bertholletiae/polymorpha* isolate, including toxin biodegradation by-products, was done through analysis on LC/MS-ToF 6230 (Agilent Technologies Inc., USA) and analytical standard as well as profile data as per [31, 35] using a mycotoxin/biodegradation by-product database, with the assumption that samples were assumed to lose an electron with the H^+ proton being hypothetically the lost ion. Compounds were initially mined based on their molecular features and verified by mining based on their exact formulas. The extracted ion chromatogram (EIC) of matched compounds is presented in **Supplementary Figure 2**.

3. Proposed mitigation strategy

3.1 *N. mirabilis* extracts collection, characterisation and application

The assessment of the physicochemical characteristics of the *N. mirabilis* pitcher juice used was similar to that in [36–38]. Thus, the assessment revealed the following: conductivity: 5.89 S/m, redox potential: 510 mV, specific gravity (SG): 1.02 and a pH of 2.5.

Additionally, a qualitative method for the analysis and enzymes/biochemical tests were done to determine the presence of enzymes in the pitcher juice [36–39]. Furthermore, the VITEK 2 DensiChek™ cards were used (as a supplementary method) to quantitatively determine the enzyme presence in the extracts during the physicochemical analysis of the pitcher juice according to the instrument's/device's user manual instructions [40].

3.2 Enzyme (carboxylesterase) activity: mechanism, specificity and quantification

The quantification of carboxylesterases activity was similar to the method adopted from [41–43] with minor modifications. The overall biocatalysis properties of the *N. mirabilis* pitcher constituents, with a focus on carboxylesterases, are described by [41], who suggested that hydrolysis mechanism associated with carboxylesterases facilitates the biocatalysis of reactions associated with enzymes, including arylesterase, lysophospholipase, acetylesterase, acylglycerol lipase, etc. In the current study, the biodegradation of fumonisin and deoxynivalenol (DON) was achieved using a single enzyme (carboxylesterases).

Furthermore, subsequent reports on the development of a spectrophotometric method used for the determination of carboxylesterase activity for the *N. mirabilis* digestive fluid were used by [29, 42].

3.3 Carboxylesterase activity assay

Previous studies assessed carboxylesterase activity. Thus, the carboxylesterase activity assay was determined spectrophotometrically at an ambient temperature using *p*-nitrophenyl acetate (PNPA) as the substrate as suggested by [36, 43]. While the activity was measured by determining the rate of biocatalysis of PNPA to *p*-nitrophenol (PNP) which was spectrophotometrically monitored at 410 nm. The PNPA exhibits minimal absorbance at 410 nm, whereas the PNP absorbs strongly. The extinction coefficient used for PNP was 17,000 $M^{-1}\cdot cm^{-1}$ [36]. Activity was then expressed in U/L, where 1 unit is equivalent to 1 μmol/min (the rate of conversion for PNPA to PNP).

3.4 Spectrophotometer settings: Carboxylesterase activity assay

The JENWAY 6405 UV/Vis spectrophotometer (Agilent Pty, USA) at a kinetics setting was used 410 nm to monitor PNP formation for 2 min at 10 sec intervals, while the cell holder temperature was at 25°C. Eq. (1) Illustrates the mathematical expression used to quantify the activity of carboxylesterases [36].

$$\text{activity } (\text{U}/\text{L}) = \left[\frac{\frac{dA}{dt} * (\text{dilution factor})}{\text{extinction coefficient}} \right] * 60 * 10^6 \tag{1}$$

Where $\frac{dA}{dt}$ is the value of the reaction's initial rate.

4. Mycotoxins identification

Mycotoxins produced by the isolated *C. bertholletiae/polymorpha* were assessed via a fermentation technique in a nutrient broth medium with the liquid-liquid extraction method being done using chloroform, subsequent to a blow-down technique of the samples and reconstitution in absolute methanol. The compounds listed in **Table 1** were identified based on their molecular composition (structural features) and mass-to-charge ratio (*m/z*), using an LC/MS-ToF.

Toxin identification is important due to observed consequential outcomes of the infested cassava as by-products of bacterial or mycotic infestation which are hazardous to both humans and animals if such agricultural product is consumed. Thus, both fumonisin B[1] and deoxynivalenol were identified as the prevalent compounds associated with the fermentation of the cyanide resistant isolate, *C. bertholletiae*, accession no. KT275316 [15].

FB[1] detection on LC/MS-ToF was done, based on a method developed by [18, 24, 31, 44], for which the analyte produces a signal under a positive MS acquisition mode (**Table 1**).

A, mycotoxins molar mass (g/mol); B, biodegradation by-products molar mass (g/mol); A1, mycotoxins mass (*m/z*) to charge ratio-ion form $[M + H]^+$; B1, biodegradation by-products mass (*m/z*) to charge ratio-ion form.

For FB[1], mean peak counts of 4×10^3 were observed, while 1.9×10^3 counts were for DON. Similarly, and according to [31], DON detection is easily achieved through HPLC/LC-MS and UV methods. A LC/MS–ToF method, as described above, was used without modification nor optimisation, to also identify the biodegradation by-products for each identified mycotoxins/secondary metabolite as listed in **Table 1**.

Two peaks were observed with a retention time of 23.79 and 35.12 min, with a molecular formula of $C_{34}H_{59}NO_{15}$ and $C_{15}H_{20}O_6$, analogous to FB[1] and DON, respectively. The peaks, A and B, were directly associated with ion *m/z* of 722.395 and 297.13, when the ESI was operated in a positive mode [ion form: $M + H^+$]. From the analysis, a combination of the molecular weight, the structure, including *m/z* ratio, confirmed the identification of the compounds. It is paramount to indicate that FB[1] was detected in a culture in which CN^- (as KCN) was supplemented; hypothetically, indicating that the FB[1] production was perhaps influenced by strenuous conditions to which the culture was subjected in comparison to DON.

4.1 Biodegradation by-products' identification

To the reported residual samples of the cyanide-resistant *C. bertholletiaee/polymorpha*, in which FB[1] and DON were detected, *N. mirabilis* pitcher juices were added. This was for an assessment of the fungal mycotoxins/toxins' (FB[1] and DON) biodegradation into by-products [36–38], which could be identified using the LC/MS-ToF. Thus, compounds such as heptadecanone, octadecanamide and octadecenal were successfully identified from FB[1] samples with only 3-keto-DON being identified in DON samples, respectively (**Table 1**; **Figure 1**).

Mycotoxins/secondary metabolites	Biodegradation by-products identified	Molar mass (g/mol)		(*m/z*) ion form $[M + H]^+$	
		A	B	A1	B1
Fumonisin B[1] ($C_{34}H_{59}NO_{15}$	Heptadecanone $C_{17}H_{34}O$	721	254.45	722.395	256.270
	Octadecanamide $C_{18}H_{37}NO$		283.29		284.282
	Octadecenal $C_{18}H_{34}O$		266.46		267.268
Deoxynivalenol (DON) ($C_{15}H_{20}O_6$)	3-keto-DON $C_{15}H_{18}O_6$	296	294.91	297.13	295.115

Table 1.
C. bertholletiae's *mycotoxins/toxins and mycotoxins biodegradation by-products identified using LC/MS-ToF.*

The findings of this study are similar to those from previous studies which revealed that a biodegradation of FB[1] yielded by-products such as heptadecanone, octadecanamide and octadecenal (**Supplementary Figure 2a–c**) [26, 45]. While a degradation of DON led to an intermediate by-product such as 3-keto-DON [46, 47] (**Supplementary Figure 2d**). By using a similar identification strategy to that used to identify FB[1] and DON, it was clear that *N. mirabilis* had a deleterious effect on both DON and FB[1]. The findings of this study are in agreement with those by [38, 48]. From the spectra, the by-product counts indicated octadecenal (1.1×10^2) > octadecanamide (1×10^2) > heptadecanone (0.9×10^2) with molecular ion peaks at *m/z* [$M + H^+$], 267.268, 284.282 and 256.270, respectively.

Furthermore, for DON residual samples, the by-products observed when subjected to the *N. mirabilis* pitcher juice were indicative of 3-keto-DON; that is, with the ESI spectra showing a molecular ion peak at *m/z* [$M + H^+$], 295.115 in a positive ion mode which was consistent with the molecular formula ($C_{15}H_{18}O_6$) (see **Supplementary Figure 2d**). Due to the nature of the proposed *in-situ* mitigation strategy, it is prudent to indicate that the applied *N. mirabilis* pitcher juice comprises biocatalytic agents or enzymes [39, 49] known to facilitate the

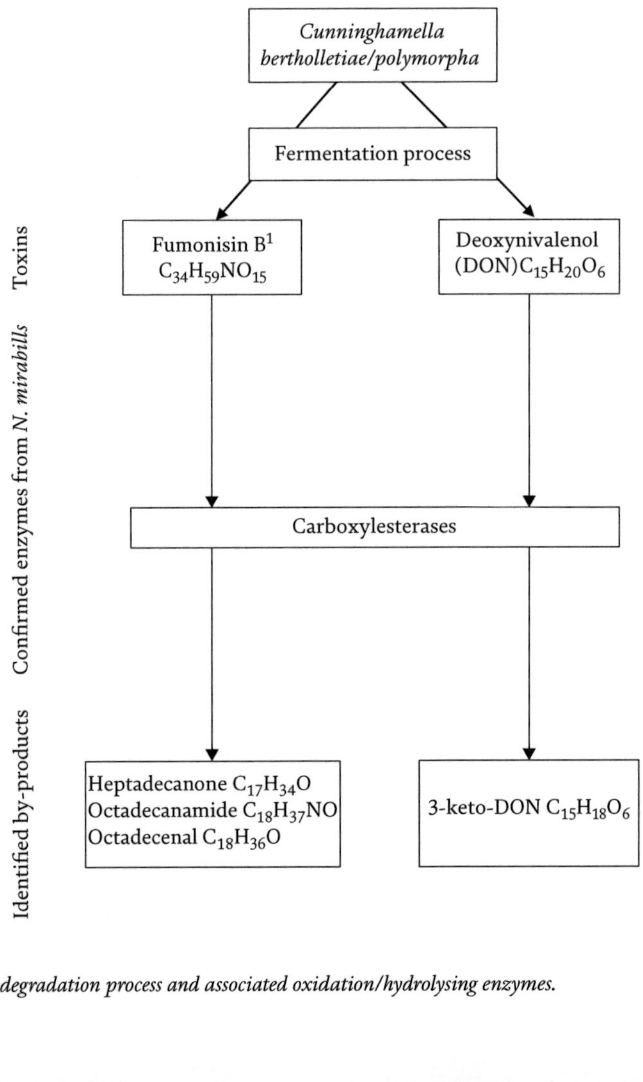

Figure 1.
Summary of a biodegradation process and associated oxidation/hydrolysing enzymes.

biodegradation of mycotoxins, using both qualitative and quantitative techniques. Thus, a degrading ability of the pitcher juice is due to the presence of enzymes such as carboxylesterase, β-glucuronidase, phosphatidyl inositol phospholipase C, xylanases, etc., which are able to biodegrade several organic matters, i.e. agro-waste, hemicellulose, etc., as well as mycotoxins/toxins [36–39, 49–51]. The enzymes found in the *N. mirabilis* pitcher juice originate from decayed multitude of trapped preys/species (insects) and microbial community (fungal and bacterial, etc.) within the plant's fluid [28, 37, 39, 41, 49, 51, 52].

4.2 Enzyme/biochemical activity assays for *N. mirabilis* pitcher juice

The samples' carboxylesterase activity (quantitative) and other biochemical assays (using the VITEK system, qualitative) were also done at room temperatures, whereas the *N. mirabilis* pitcher juice for carboxylesterase, *P*-nitrophenyl acetate (PNPA) were used as a substrate at 75% dilution and 410 nm absorbance which was similar to [36, 37]. For biochemical assays, numerous enzymes (as highlighted in **Table 2**) were positively identified, while the calculation of carboxylesterase activity was found to be 7.8 U/L.

5. Mycotoxin identification from cyanide-resistant *Cunninghamella* spp.

Due to the multitude of methods developed and assessed, a method modified by [44], for toxin extraction from a fermentation of broth, was adopted. It was thus used to produce mycotoxins (FB1 and DON) from the cyanide-resistant *C. bertholletiae/polymorpha*, with the extracts being used for LC/MS-ToF analysis due to the method's usability, reproducibility and rapidity, while incurring minimal input/sample-processing costs.

5.1 Biodegradation by-products: outcomes of the mitigation strategy

A digestive fluid of *N. mirabilis* was used as a feasible alternative for the biodegradation of fungal mycotoxins/toxins (Fumonisin and DON) with assays (n = 2) confirming the prevalence of carboxylesterases. However, previous studies mentioned the existence of several enzymes [28, 39, 41, 49, 50] within a *N. mirabilis* digestive fluid/pitcher juice, which counts as a larger enzymatic profile than individual microbial species, as highlighted in **Table 2**.

Furthermore, a few sceptics could express concern about the use of a plant's pitcher juice on mycotoxin-contaminated matrices because of its low pH (2.5), as well as availability, which can be addressed by using appropriate buffers and suitable plant

Enzymes	Activity/outcome	References
Carboxylesterase	7.8 (U/L)	In this study
β-glucosidase	++	[38, 39]
β-glucuronidase	++	[48]
Phosphatidyl inositol phospholipase C	++	[49]

++, positively identified in previous studies.

Table 2.
Carboxylesterase activity and qualitatively identified enzymes.

extracts with similar enzymatic characteristics. Overall, the application of a low pH extract in a matrix such as agricultural soil should not be a major concern because a soil's pH can be amended by an application of lime. A study by [53] revealed that the application of lime on agricultural soil with a low pH increases the soil's pH, improving its respiration capacity, while retaining the soil's microbial community profile at an acceptable level.

6. Conclusions

The identification through LC/MS-ToF of toxins ((fumonisin B^1 and deoxynivalenol (DON)) from a free-cyanide-resistant *Cunninghamella bertholletiae/polymorpha* as well as a mitigation strategy for toxins reduction through a biodegradation/fermentation process using 'monkey cup' juice from *N. mirabilis* (which yielded by-products such as heptadecanone, octadecanamide, octadecenal and 3-keto-DON) is an important step towards ensuring food safety and mitigating humans' health hazards through toxins exposure. As, an exposure or intoxication from these mycotoxins, through consumption of contaminated food or agricultural product, can be hazardous to humans and animals. Therefore, control measures for food and animal feed contamination are needed in order to decrease the levels of these compounds. Additionally, preventative protocols and/or mitigation strategies that would ensure the eradication of these hazardous compounds, using an environmentally benign approach such as *N. mirabilis* digestive fluid/pitcher juices, are paramount. Thus, the application of the digestive fluid to a liquid matrix which culminated in the biodegradation of mycotoxins (fumonisin B1 and DON), with the subsequent formation of the biodegradation by-products such as heptadecanone, octadecanamide, octadecenal for fumonisin B1 and 3-keto-DON for DON, which are easier to biodegrade by other microbial communities, should be encouraged.

However, it is worth noting that at this stage, there is a need to find alternative indigenous plant extracts with similar characteristics to that of the *N. mirabilis*.

Acknowledgements

The authors would like to express their gratitude to: Ogheneochuko Oputu, all BioERG members as well as staff from the Environmental Management Programme and Biotechnology department for their support.

Funding

The research is funded by the Cape Peninsula University of Technology, through the University Research Fund (URF)—Cost code R980.

Conflicts of interest

The authors declare no conflicts of interest with respect to the research, authorship and/or publication of this manuscript.

Appendix

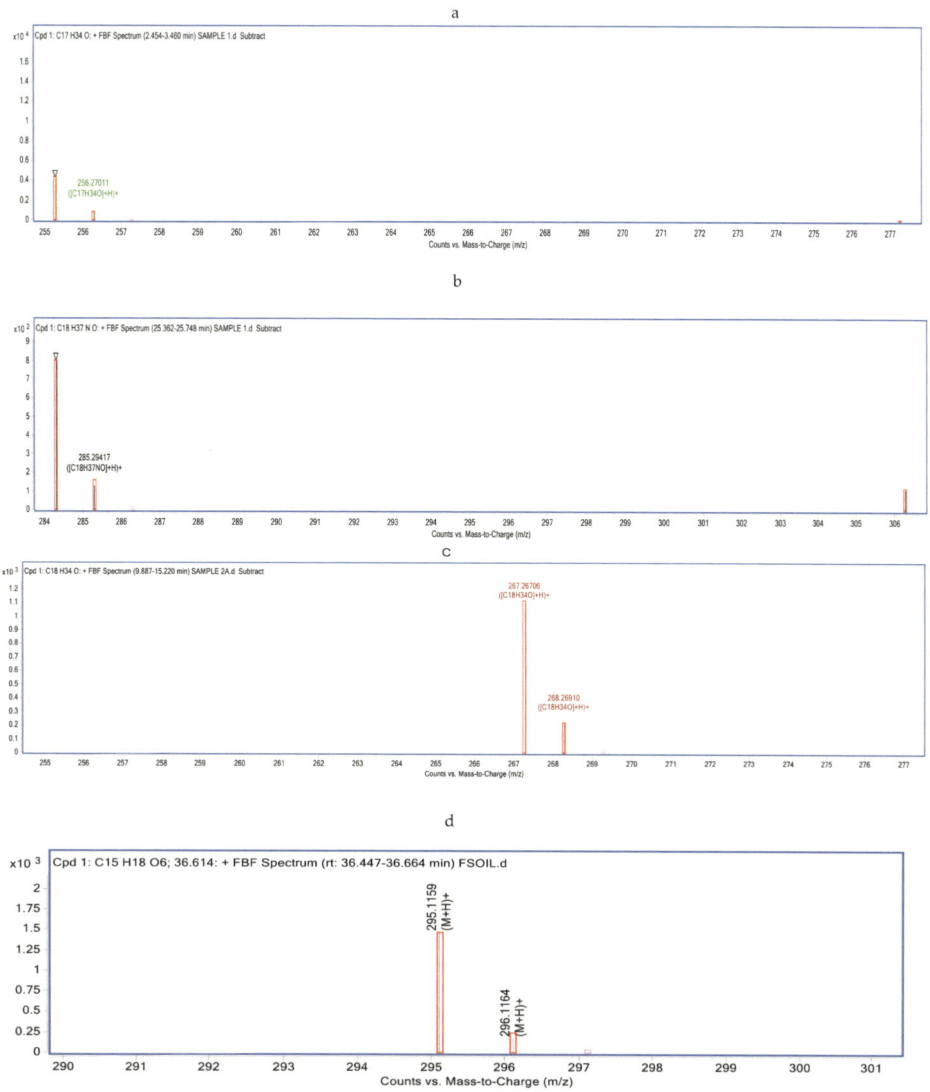

Supplementary Figure 2.
Molecular features and the extracted ion chromatograms (EICs)/mass spectrum of mycotoxins/toxins' biodegradation by-products: (a) heptadecanone, (b) octadecanamide, (c) octadecenal and (d) 3-keto-DON.

Gradient (min)	A (H_2O)*	B (MeOH)Y	Flow (mL/min)
0	85	15	0.4
30	0	100	0.4
33	0	100	0.4
45	85	15	0.4
50	85	15	0.4

**, water contained, 0.1% formic acid, pH 3.*
Y, analytical grade methanol.

Supplementary Table S1.
LC/MS-ToF elution and mobile phase parameters.

Author details

Elie Fereche Itoba-Tombo[1*], Seteno Karabo Obed Ntwampe[2], John Baptist Nzukizi Mudumbi[3], Lukhanyo Mekuto[4], Enoch Akinbiyi Akinpelu[3] and Nkosikho Dlangamandla[5]

1 Department of Environmental and Occupational Studies, Cape Peninsula University of Technology, Cape Town, South Africa

2 School of Chemical and Mineral Engineering, North-West University, Potchefstroom, South Africa

3 Bioresource Engineering Research Group (BioERG), Department of Biotechnology, Cape Peninsula University of Technology, Cape Town, South Africa

4 Department of Chemical Engineering, University of Johannesburg, Johannesburg, South Africa

5 Department of Chemical Engineering, Durban University of Technology, Durban, South Africa

*Address all correspondence to: elie.tombo@gmail.com

References

[1] Pitt JI, Hocking AD. The ecology of fungal food spoilage. In: Pitt JI, Hocking AD, editors. Fungi and Food Spoilage. Boston, MA: Springer; 2009. pp. 3-9

[2] Zidenga T, Leyva-Guerrero E, Moon H, Siritunga D, Sayre R. Extending cassava root shelf life via reduction of reactive oxygen species production. Plant Physiology. 2012;**159**:1396-1407

[3] Matumba L, Sulyok M, Monjerezi M, Biswick T, Krska R. Fungal metabolites diversity in maize and associated human dietary exposures relate to micro-climatic patterns in Malawi. World Mycotoxin Journal. 2014;**8**(3):269-282

[4] Weitzman I, Crist MY. Studies with clinical isolates of *Cunninghamella* I. Mating behavior. Mycologia. 1979;**71**:1024-1033

[5] Wagacha J, Muthomi J. Mycotoxin problem in Africa: Current status, implications to food safety and health and possible management strategies. International Journal of Food Microbiology. 2008;**124**(1):1-12

[6] Nguyen TT, Choi YJ, Lee HB. Isolation and characterization of three unrecorded zygomycete fungi in Korea: *Cunninghamella bertholletiae*, *Cunninghamella echinulata*, and *Cunninghamella elegan*. Mycobiology. 2017;**45**(4):318-326

[7] Zhang R, Zhang JW, Szerlip HM. Endocarditis and hemorrhagic stroke caused by *Cunninghamella bertholletiae* infection after kidney transplantation. American Journal of Kidney Diseases. 2002;**40**(4):842-846

[8] Ueno Y, Iijima K, Wang SD, Sugiura Y, Sekijima M, Tanaka T, et al. Fumonisins as a possible contributory risk factor for primary liver cancer: A 3-year study of corn harvested in Haimen, China, by HPLC and ELISA. Food and Chemical Toxicology. 1997;**35**(12):1143-1150

[9] Brakhage AA. Regulation of fungal secondary metabolism. Nature Reviews Microbiology. 2013;**11**(1):21-32

[10] Selvaraj JN, Lu Z, Yan W, Zhao YJ, Xing FG, Dai XF, et al. Mycotoxin detection—Recent trends at global level. Journal of Integrative Agriculture. 2015;**14**(11):2265-2281

[11] Amadi JE, Adeniyi DO. Mycotoxin production by fungi isolated from stored grains. African Journal of Biotechnology. 2009;**8**(7):1219-1221

[12] Adetunji M, Atanda O, Ezekiel CN, Sulyok M, Warth B, Beltrán E, et al. Fungal and bacterial metabolites of stored maize (*Zea mays*) from five agro-ecological zones of Nigeria. Mycotoxin Research. 2014;**30**(2):89-102

[13] Delgado RM, Sulyok M, Jirsa O, Spitzer T, Krska R, Polišenská I. Relationship between lutein and mycotoxin content in durum wheat. Food Additives & Contaminants: Part A. 2014;**31**(7):1274-1283

[14] Njumbe Ediage E, Hell K, De Saeger S. A comprehensive study to explore differences in mycotoxin patterns from agro-ecological regions through maize, peanut, and cassava products: A case study, Cameroon. Journal of Agricultural and Food Chemistry. 2014;**62**(20):4789-4797

[15] Itoba-Tombo EF, Waxa A, Ntwampe SKO. Isolation of an endophytic cyanide resistant fungus

Cunninghamella bertholletiae from (*Manihot esculenta*) and cassava cultivated soil for environmental engineering applications. In: 7th International Conference on Latest Trends in Engineering and Technology (ICLTET'2015); 26-27 November 2015; Pretoria, South Africa. 2015. pp. 150-153

[16] Itoba-Tombo EF, Ntwampe SKO, Mudumbi JBN, Mekuto L, Akinpelu EA, Oputu OU. Rapid identification of *Cunninghamella bertholletiae*'s toxins/ secondary metabolites via a fermentation technique. In: 10th Int'l Conference on Advances in Chemical, Agricultural, Biological and Environmental Sciences (ACABES-18); 19-20 November 2018; Cape Town, South Africa. 2018 [Retrieved: 17 September 2018]

[17] Streit E, Schwab C, Sulyok M, Naehrer K, Krska R, Schatzmayr G. Multi-mycotoxin screening reveals the occurrence of 139 different secondary metabolites in feed and feed ingredients. Toxins. 2013;**5**(3):504-523

[18] Warth B, Petchkongkaew A, Sulyok M, Krska R. Utilising an LC-MS/MS-based multi-biomarker approach to assess mycotoxin exposure in the Bangkok metropolitan area and surrounding provinces. Food Additives & Contaminants: Part A. 2014;**31**(12):2040-2046

[19] Mantle P, Copetti MV, Buddie A, Frisvad J. Comments on "Mycobiota and Mycotoxins in Traditional Medicinal Seeds from China. Toxins 2015, 7, 3858-3875"—In attributing ochratoxin A biosynthesis within the genus *Penicillium* occurring on natural agricultural produce. Toxins. 2016;**8**(6):1-4

[20] Williams JH, Phillips TD, Jolly PE, Stiles JK, Jolly CM, Aggarwal D. Human aflatoxicosis in developing countries: A review of toxicology, exposure, potential health consequences, and interventions. The American Journal of Clinical Nutrition. 2004;**80**(5):1106-1122

[21] Pestka JJ, Smolinski AT. Deoxynivalenol: toxicology and potential effects on humans. Journal of Toxicology and Environmental Health, Part B. 2005;**8**(1):39-69

[22] Afsah-Hejri L, Jinap S, Hajeb P, Radu S, Shakibazadeh S. A review on mycotoxins in food and feed: Malaysia case study. Comprehensive Reviews in Food Science and Food Safety. 2013;**12**(6):629-651

[23] Rickerts V, Böhme A, Viertel A, Behrendt G, Jacobi V, Tintelnot K, et al. Cluster of pulmonary infections caused by *Cunninghamella bertholletiae* in immunocompromised patients. Clinical Infectious Diseases. 2000;**31**(4):910-913

[24] Srey C, Kimanya ME, Routledge MN, Shirima CP, Gong YY. Deoxynivalenol exposure assessment in young children in Tanzania. Molecular Nutrition & Food Research. 2014;**58**(7):1574-1580

[25] Van Der Fels-Klerx HJ, Olesen JE, Madsen MS, Goedhart PW. Climate change increases deoxynivalenol contamination of wheat in north-western Europe. Food Additives & Contaminants: Part A. 2012;**29**(10):1593-1604

[26] Vanhoutte I, Audenaert K, De Gelder L. Biodegradation of mycotoxins: Tales from known and unexplored worlds. Frontiers in Microbiology. 2016;7:1-20

[27] Itoba-Tombo EF, Ntwampe SKO, Waxa A, Paulse A, Akinpelu EA. Screening of fungal (*Cunnighamella bertholletiae*) pathogenic activity on microbial community in cassava (*Manihot esculenta crantz*) cultivated soil. In: Int'l Conf. on Advances in Science,

Engineering, Technology and Natural Resources (ICASETNR-16); 24-25 November 2016; Parys, South Africa. 2016. pp. 112-117

[28] Adlassnig W, Peroutka M, Lendl T. Traps of carnivorous pitcher plants as a habitat: Composition of the fluid, biodiversity and mutualistic activities. Annals of Botany. 2010;**107**(2):181-194

[29] Lee L, Zhang Y, Ozar B, Sensen CW, Schriemer DC. Carnivorous nutrition in pitcher plants (*Nepenthes* spp.) via an unusual complement of endogenous enzymes. Journal of Proteome Research. 2016;**15**(9):3108-3117

[30] Peraica M, Domijan AM. Contamination of food with mycotoxins and human health. Arhiv za Higijenu Rada i Toksikologiju. 2001;**52**(1):23-35

[31] Sulyok M, Beed F, Boni S, Abass A, Mukunzi A, Krska R. Quantitation of multiple mycotoxins and cyanogenic glucosides in cassava samples from Tanzania and Rwanda by an LC-MS/MS-based multi-toxin method. Food Additives & Contaminants: Part A. 2015;**32**(4):488-502

[32] Rubert J, Soler C, Marín R, James KJ, Mañes J. Mass spectrometry strategies for mycotoxins analysis in European beers. Food Control. 2013;**30**(1):122-128

[33] Lattanzio VMT, Solfrizzo M, Powers S, Visconti A. Simultaneous determination of aflatoxins, ochratoxin A and *Fusarium* toxins in maize by liquid chromatography/tandem mass spectrometry after multitoxin immunoaffinity cleanup. Rapid Communications in Mass Spectrometry. 2007;**21**(20):3253-3261

[34] Farag MA, Porzel A, Wessjohann LA. Comparative metabolite profiling and fingerprinting of medicinal licorice roots using a multiplex approach of GC–MS, LC–MS and 1D NMR techniques. Phytochemistry. 2012;**76**:60-72

[35] Zide D, Fatoki O, Oputu O, Opeolu B, Nelana S, Olatunji O. Zeolite 'adsorption' capacities in aqueous acidic media; the role of acid choice and quantification method on ciprofloxacin removal. Microporous and Mesoporous Materials. 2018;**255**:226-241

[36] Dlangamandla N, Ntwampe SKO, Angadam JO, Chidi BS, Mewa-Ngongang M. Kinetic parameters of *Saccharomyces cerevisiae* alcohols production using *Nepenthes mirabilis* pod digestive fluids-mixed agro-waste hydrolysates. Fermentation. 2019;**1**(5):1-14

[37] Dlangamandla N, Ntwampe SKO, Angadam JO, Itoba-Tombo EF, Chidi BS, Mekuto L. Integrated hydrolysis of mixed agro-waste for a second generation biorefinery using *Nepenthes mirabilis* pod digestive fluids. PRO. 2019;**7**(2):64

[38] Kanokratana P, Mhuanthong W, Laothanachareon T, Tangphatsornruang S, Eurwilaichitr L, Kruetreepradit T, et al. Comparative study of bacterial communities in *Nepenthes pitchers* and their correlation to species and fluid acidity. Microbial Ecology. 2016;**72**(2):381-393

[39] Takeuchi Y, Salcher MM, Ushio M, Shimizu-Inatsugi R, Kobayashi MJ, Diway B, et al. In-situ enzyme activity in the dissolved and particulate fraction of the fluid from four pitcher plant species of the genus *Nepenthes*. PLoS One. 2011;**6**(9):1-9

[40] Pincus DH. Microbial Identification Using the Bio Merieux VITEK® 2 System. Encyclopedia of Rapid Microbiological Methods. Bethesda, MD: Parenteral Drug Association; 2006

[41] Schomburg D. Brenda. The comprehensive enzyme information system (online). 2015. Available from: http://www.brenda-enzymes.org/enzyme.php [Retrieved: 10 October 2018]

[42] Wheelock CE, Severson TF, Hammock BD. Synthesis of new carboxylesterase inhibitors and evaluation of potency and water solubility. Chemical Research in Toxicology. 2001;**14**(12):1563-1572

[43] Ljungquist A, Augustinsson KB. Purification and properties of two carboxylesterases from rat-liver microsomes. European Journal of Biochemistry. 1971;**23**(2):303-313

[44] Bily AC, Burt AJ, Ramputh AI, Livesey J, Regnault-Roger C, Philogène BR, et al. HPLC-PAD-APCI/MS assay of phenylpropanoids in cereals. Phytochemical Analysis. 2004;**15**(1):9-15

[45] Benedetti R, Nazzi F, Locci R, Firrao G. Degradation of fumonisin B1 by a bacteria strain isolated from soil. Biodegradation. 2006;**17**(1):31-38

[46] He JW, Bondy GS, Zhou T, Caldwell D, Boland GJ, Scott PM. Toxicology of 3-epi-deoxynivalenol, a deoxynivalenol-transformation product by *Devosia mutans* 17-2-E-8. Food and Chemical Toxicology. 2015;**84**:250-259

[47] He JW, Hassan YI, Perilla N, Li XZ, Boland GJ, Zhou T. Bacterial epimerization as a route for deoxynivalenol detoxification: The influence of growth and environmental conditions. Frontiers in Microbiology. 2016a;**7**:572

[48] Duvick J, Maddox J, Gilliam J. Compositions and methods for fumonisin detoxification. U.S. Patent No. 6,538,177. Pioneer Hi-Bred International Inc.; 2003

[49] Terra WR, Ferreira C. Insect digestive enzymes: Properties, compartmentalization and function. Comparative Biochemistry and Physiology Part B: Comparative Biochemistry. 1994;**109**(1):1-62

[50] Borgen BH. Functional analysis of plant idioblasts (myrosin cells) and their role in defense, development and growth. In: Thesis Submitted for the degree of Doctor Scientiarum at the Norwegian University of Science and Technology (NTNU). UNIGEN Center of Molecular Biology and Department of Biology, Faculty of Natural Sciences and Technology; 2002

[51] Hassan YI, He JW, Perilla N, Tang K, Karlovsky P, Zhou T. The enzymatic epimerization of deoxynivalenol by *Devosia mutans* proceeds through the formation of 3-keto-DON intermediate. Scientific Reports. 2017;**7**:6929

[52] Carere J, Hassan YI, Lepp D, Zhou T. The enzymatic detoxification of the mycotoxin deoxynivalenol: Identification of DepA from the DON epimerization pathway. Microbial Biotechnology. 2018;**11**(6):1106-1111

[53] Bezdicek DF, Beaver T, Granatstein D. Subsoil ridge tillage and lime effects on soil microbial activity, soil pH, erosion, and wheat and pea yield in the Pacific Northwest, USA. Soil and Tillage Research. 2003;**74**(1):55-63

Chapter 7

Mycotoxin Decontamination of Foods Using Nonthermal Plasma and Plasma-Activated Water

Hsiu-Ling Chen, Rachelle D. Arcega, Samuel Herianto, Chih-Yao Hou and Chia-Min Lin

Abstract

Mycotoxins are food safety and public health concerns due to their widespread contamination in agricultural products and adverse health effects on humans. Several decontamination techniques, including physical-, chemical-, and thermal-based treatments, are employed to minimize the levels of mycotoxins in food. However, these treatments present disadvantages, such as negative impacts on the quality and leftover chemical residues on the treated food after physical- and chemical-based treatments. Furthermore, mycotoxins are resistant to heat, thus contributing to the insufficiency of thermal treatments for complete mycotoxin degradation. The use of alternative nonthermal-based treatments, such as nonthermal plasma (NTP) and plasma-activated water (PAW) for mycotoxin degradation in food, have been recently explored to overcome these limitations. NTP and PAW treatments are known to minimize the unfavorable changes in food quality while ensuring safety from food contaminants. The basics of NTP and PAW technologies, their mycotoxin decontamination efficiencies, their underlying mechanisms of action, effects on food quality, and the safety of mycotoxin degradation byproducts and treated food are hereby discussed in this chapter.

Keywords: mycotoxin, nonthermal plasma, plasma-activated water, mechanism of action, food quality, toxicity

1. Introduction

Mycotoxins are naturally occurring toxins or secondary metabolites produced by a wide range of fungal species (molds), including *Aspergillus*, *Claviceps*, *Fusarium*, *Penicillium*, and *Alternaria* [1]. These microorganisms usually colonize in crops and plants; thus, they can release the mycotoxin compounds and further contaminate the agricultural products during pre-harvest, harvest, and post-harvest [2]. Enyiukwu et al. [3] reported that approximately 25% of the global food and feed output is contaminated by mycotoxins. Furthermore, researchers have identified around 300 types of mycotoxins and revealed that 10 of these toxic compounds, such as aflatoxins, ochratoxins, zearalenone (ZEN), ergotamine, deoxynivalenol (DON), fumonisins, nivalenol, enniatin, citrinin, and trichothecenes, commonly contaminate agriculture-based foods worldwide [4]. These molecules can induce mycotoxicosis (acute and chronic toxic diseases) in humans, raising concerns toward food safety and public health [1]. Additionally, mycotoxin contaminations have been reported to be responsible for significant economic losses [4]. For instance, the costs for the agricultural industry or food supply chain induced by mycotoxin contamination are USD 1.5 billion/year in the United States [5].

Multiple methods, ranging from conventional-, physical-, to chemical-based treatments, have been employed throughout the years to detoxify and decontaminate mycotoxin from agricultural products. The conventional approaches, including cooking and pasteurization, are simple and low-cost treatments; however, several mycotoxins can resist such thermal-based treatments [6]. Meanwhile, physical and chemical approaches, such as microwave [7], ozone [8], essential oils [9], and pulsed light irradiation [10], have been widely applied. However, these typical treatments are still problematic because they may result in undesirable changes in the physical, chemical, and sensory properties of the treated foods.

Nonthermal-based treatments, such as nonthermal plasma (NTP) and plasma-activated water (PAW), have recently gained considerable attention in food safety because they possess significant antimicrobial capacity against a wide range of food-borne pathogens without negative effects on food quality [11, 12]. Gaseous NTP and PAW richly contain multiple charged particles, reactive oxygen species (ROS), and reactive nitrogen species (RNS); thus, these methods have been proposed to prevent the risk of mycotoxin contaminations in various foods [4]. Ultimately, the effectiveness of both systems has rapid growth for decontaminating multiple foods from various microorganisms, such as *Saccharomyces cerevisiae*, *Escherichia coli*, *Staphylococcus aureus*, *Bacillus cereus*, *Klebsiella pneumonia*, and *Listeria monocytogenes*, as widely reviewed by Herianto et al. [11], Perinban et al. [13], Thirumdas et al. [14], and Zhou et al. [15]. Nevertheless, a review focusing on their effects on mycotoxin deactivations is unavailable. Thus, this chapter briefly discusses the applications of NTP and PAW for mycotoxin decontamination in various agricultural foods and their respective effects on food quality according to the most up-to-date studies. In addition, the decontamination mechanism of reactive species by both systems over mycotoxin is elaborated. Finally, constructive suggestions are also provided to stimulate satisfactory research of this field in the future.

2. Fundamentals of NTP and PAW

NTP represents a physical agent compromising a mixture of charged particles, neutral particles, radicals, ultraviolet (UV) radiation, and reactive species (RNS and ROS), which can induce oxidative stress and death of cells or organisms upon interactions [16]. Electrical energy is normally used to introduce feeding gases, such as ambient air, argon (Ar), helium (He), and oxygen (O_2), into the plasma phase to form NTP, which further generates a combination of the above-mentioned species [17]. Plasma can be effectively generated through the following four main systems of devices—electric arc discharges, corona discharges, plasma jet, and dielectric barrier discharges (DBD) [13]. Among these configuration systems, plasma jet and DBD are preferred due to their simplicity and efficient capability of producing richly reactive species [11]. Particularly, plasma jet utilizes discharged plasma electrodes that can extend beyond the area of plasma generation into the surrounding ambiance [18], further facilitating an effective interaction with the treated foods. Meanwhile, DBD uses discharges produced between two electrodes, which are separated by dielectric barrier materials, such as glass and ceramic [19]. Foods of interest can be placed between two electrodes for plasma exposure and treatment, further allowing for interaction and decontaminations.

Meanwhile, PAW is a liquid product of chemical reactions of NTP with water, containing a rich variety of high ROS and RNS [20]. ROS includes several chemically reactive molecules and free radicals containing molecular oxygen, such as hydrogen peroxide (H_2O_2), hydroxyl radical (•OH), ozone (O_3), superoxides (O_2^-,), singlet oxygen ($^1O_2$), and alpha-oxygen [21]. By contrast, RNS is a group of nitric oxide-derived compounds, including NO_2^-, NO_3^-, nitroxyl anion, peroxynitrite ($OONO^-$), nitrosonium cation, and S-nitrosothiols [22]. In particular, Herianto et al. [11] reviewed the detailed reaction mechanism of the formation of these reactive species. Several key parameters for performing these reactions and successful PAW generations include water sources (sterile distilled water, deionized water, reverse osmosis water, and tap water), working gas (air, Ar, He, and O_2), power, activation time, gas flow rate, and position of the plasma electrode toward water [11, 12].

Unlike NTP, as a liquid solution, PAW enables a maximal exposure of reactive species to the entire surface of the treated foods, suggesting large-scale applications over various agricultural products in large volumes [11, 20]. Overall, both systems have been successfully applied for decontaminating various foods and agricultural products, such as vegetables (baby spinach leaves, mushroom, and mung bean sprout), fruits (grape tomato, grape, Chinese bayberry, and strawberry), fresh-cut fruits and vegetables (fresh-cut apple, pear, kiwifruit, endive lettuce, celery, and radicchio), meats (beef, chicken breast), shrimps, eggs, and rice cake [11, 12, 14, 23–27]. The application of these decontamination systems for mycotoxins is discussed in Section 3.

3. Mycotoxin degradation in food using NTP and PAW

Several researchers have utilized NTP and PAW treatments for the degradation of different mycotoxins in recent years to minimize the mycotoxin levels in food [28, 29]. Two possible pathways are generally available to achieve mycotoxin degradation—(1) inactivation of the fungi that produce the mycotoxins, herein referred to as mycotoxin-producing fungi (MPF), and (2) direct degradation of the mycotoxins. The most recent findings of the studies that target the two pathways using NTP and PAW treatments are respectively presented in Sections 3.1 and 3.2.

3.1 Inactivation of MPF

The application of NTP for the inactivation of MPF in food has been comprehensively reviewed in the past [28, 30], whereas a review on the effects of PAW on MPF inactivation is still lacking. Therefore, this chapter emphasizes the key findings from the most recent NTP studies, particularly in the past 3 years, and all PAW studies, to provide updated information on the current progress of these technologies for MPF inactivation. The application of NTP and PAW is generally commonly prevalent in nuts, seeds, and spices, and the commonly challenged MPF includes species that are mainly from the *Aspergillus (A.)*, *Alternaria (Alt.),* and *Fusarium (F.)* fungal genera due to their capability to produce mycotoxins. These findings are summarized in **Table 1**.

Plasma device and treatment parameters	**Food matrix**	**MPF of concern**	**Key findings**	**Source**
a. NTP treatment				
Device: DBD Gas: ambient air Power supply: 130 W, 20 kHz, 15 kV Distance from electrode to sample: 3 mm Treatment time: 0.25, 0.50, 1, 1.50, 2, 2.50, 3 min	Pistachio nuts	*A. flavus*	• Population of viable *A. flavus* spores significantly decreased with respect to time compared to control (no treatment) • Complete inactivation of *A. flavus* after 3 min of treatment	Makari et al. [31]
Device: large-scale RF plasma system Gas: O_2 gas Gas flow rate: 202 standard mL/min Power supply: 1500 W, 27.12 mHz Treatment time: 0.25, 0.50, 0.75, 1, 1.50, 2 min	Common and Tartary buckwheat seeds	*Alternaria*, *Fusarium*	• Frequency and diversity of both fungal communities significantly reduced after 1.50 and 2 min of plasma treatment of common and Tartary buckwheat seeds, respectively	Mravlje et al. [30]
Device: planar-type DBD Gas: pure Ar, Ar/O_2 mixture at 80%/20% Gas flow rate: 1 L/min Power supply: 60 Hz, 120 V Treatment time: 10 min, once a day for 3 days	Ginseng seeds	*Fusarium*	• Survival rates of *Fusarium* were about 80 and 55% after Ar/O_2 and Ar NTP treatments, respectively	Lee et al. [32]
Devices: AP-CCP, DC-DP, ICP Gas: Ar Power supply: 50, 75, 100, 150 W (AP-CCP), 250 W (ICP), 50–300 W (DC-DP) Treatment time: 2, 6, 10 min (AP-CCP), 20 min (ICP), 5–20 min (DC-DP)	Pistachio nuts	*A. flavus*	• AP-CCP completely reduced *A. flavus* (6 log reduction) at 150 W and 10 min but produced minor alteration on pistachio shells • ICP achieved 2 log reductions at 250 W and 20 min • DC-DP achieved 5 log reductions at 300 W, 20 min, and 2 Torr pressure • Overall, AP-CCP was the optimum device when fungi inactivation and cost feasibility for large scale application were considered	Ghorashi et al. [33]

Plasma device and treatment parameters	Food matrix	MPF of concern	Key findings	Source
Device: microwave-combined cold plasma (MCP) in low- and high-density modes Gas: $He:O_2$ mixture at 99.80:0.20 Power supply: 2.45 GHz, 900 W Treatment time: 20 min	Red pepper flakes	*A. flavus*	• *A. flavus* was reduced by 1.50 and 1.60 log spores/cm^2 after low- and high-density MCP treatments, respectively, from 4.20 log spores/cm^2 and remained constant for 150 days storage at 25°C	Kim et al. [34]
Device: RDBD Gas: commercial He Gas flow rate: 1.50 L/min Power supply: 30 W, 850 V Treatment time: 0, 1, 2, 4, 5, 6, 8, 10, 12, 14, 16, 18 min	Roasted ground coffee	*A. westerdijikiae*, *A. steynii*, *A. versicolor*	• Complete inhibition of all fungal spores (4 log reductions) after 6 min of treatment	Casas-Junco et al. [35]
Device: AP and LP plasma systems Gas: N_2, air (AP); O_2, N_2, air (LP) Gas flow rate: 3000 L/h (AP) Power supply: 655 W, 25 kHz (AP); 100 W, 13.56 MHz (LP) Distance from electrode/jet to sample: 7 cm (AP); 10 cm (LP) Treatment time: 5 cycles or 1.7 min (AP); 30 min (LP)	Hazelnuts	*A. flavus*, *A. parasiticus*	• LP plasma treatment resulted in 4.40 (N_2), 4.70 (O_2), and 5.60 (air) log CFU/g reductions in *A. parasiticus*, and 4.50 (O_2), 4.60 (N_2), and 4.70 (air) log CFU/g reduction in *A. flavus* • AP plasma treatment resulted in 5 (N_2) and 5.50 (air) log CFU/g reductions in *A. parasiticus*, and 5 (N_2) and 5.40 (air) log CFU/g reductions in *A. flavus*	Sen et al. [36]
b. PAW treatment				
Device: single-phase GAD Gas: air Gas flow rate: 7.33 dm^3/min Water source: distilled water (20 mL) Power supply: 40 VA apparent power, 50 Hz, 680 V PAW activation time: 5, 10, 20 min Treatment time: 5, 10, 20 min	Beetroot and carrot seeds	Beetroot seeds: *Alt. alternata*, *A. niger*, *F. solani*, *P. expansum*, *P. nigricans* Carrot seeds: *Alt. alternata*, *Alt. radicina*, *A. niger*, *F. avenaceum*, *P. expansum*	• PAW characteristics (20 min activation): H_2O_2 = 12 μM NO_2^- = 2.90 mM pH = 3.30 • PAW treatments resulted in either a decrease or increase in fungal colonies depending on treatment duration • PAW generally resulted in a weaker fungal decontamination effect compared to chemical treatment using sodium hypochlorite	Terebun et al. [37]

Plasma device and treatment parameters	Food matrix	MPF of concern	Key findings	Source
Device: ESDP Gas: Ar/air mixture Gas flow rate: 2 L/min Water source: DI water (50 mL) Power supply: 1.50 W/cm^2, 1 kHz PAW activation time: 20 min Treatment time: 0, 20, 40, 60 min	Chinese kale seeds	*Alt. brassicicola*	• PAW characteristics: pH = 3.50 EC^a = 130 µS/cm ORP^b = 500 mV • ESDP treatment reduced *Alt. brassicicola* by ~70% after 60 min	Suwannarat et al. [38]

[a] *Electrical conductivity.*
[b] *Oxidation-reduction potential.*

Table 1.
Recent findings on the effects of gaseous NTP and PAW treatments on the inactivation of MPF in food.

These studies revealed that NTP can achieve 100% inactivation of MPF in food, particularly of the *Aspergillus* species, which can produce the most toxic mycotoxins, that is, the aflatoxins. For example, *A. flavus* populations in pistachio nuts were completely inactivated in only 3 min of NTP treatment operated in DBD using ambient air [31]. Similarly, an atmospheric pressure capacitive coupled plasma (AP-CCP) also demonstrated complete inactivation of *A. flavus* in pistachio nuts but only after a long treatment period of 10 min using Ar gas [33]. The said study compared three different kinds of NTP treatment, which includes AP-CCP, and found that AP-CCP was the optimum device due to its most effective MPF inactivation capability and lesser cost requirements compared with direct-current diode plasma (DC-DP) and inductively coupled plasma (ICP) systems [33]. Furthermore, some food crops can be a host to multiple MPF, thus resulting in the co-occurrence of MPF in food. A study also revealed that NTP treatment using a DBD reactor with radiofrequency (RF) generator (RDBD) and He as the feed gas completely inactivated the co-occurring *Aspergillus* species, including *A. westerdijikiae, A. steynii,* and *A. versicolor*, in ground coffee after 6 min [35]. Meanwhile, other studies only achieved partial inactivation of MPF but still reduced their populations significantly. For instance, Mravlje et al. [30] used a large-scale RF plasma system operating in O_2 gas and reported significant reductions in *Alternaria* and *Fusarium* fungal communities in common and Tartary buckwheat seeds in only 1.50 and 2 min of treatment, respectively. Similarly, treatment of ginseng seeds for 3 days at 10 min each day using a planar-type DBD plasma reactor also reduced *Fusarium* populations and found that using Ar as feed gas showed higher reduction compared to that when Ar/O_2 gas mixture was used [32]. Overall, the choice of plasma device, feed gas, treatment duration, type of MPF, and food matrix can affect the efficiency of NTP treatment for MPF inactivation. As an example, Sen et al. [36] reported that the use of AP plasma resulted in higher reductions of *A. flavus* and *A. parasiticus* in hazelnuts compared with low-pressure (LP) plasma using N_2 gas in both treatments. However, AP and LP plasmas achieved an almost similar inactivation of *A. parasiticus* when the air was used.

Meanwhile, the use of PAW treatment for MPF inactivation in food did not produce the best results compared with NTP treatment. PAW generated from Ar/air mixture and distilled water using an electrohydraulic streamer discharge plasma (ESDP) system inhibited *A. brassicicola* spores in Chinese kale seeds by approximately 70% but only after a long treatment period of 60 min [38]. Terebun et al. [37] also showed that PAW operated using a single-phase gliding arc reactor (GAD) at atmospheric pressure produced inconsistent levels of inactivation of several MPF in beetroot and carrot seeds, including *Alt. alternata, A. niger, F. solani, Penicillium (P.) expansum, P. nigricans, Alt. radicina,* and *F. avenaceum*, depending on the treatment duration and fungal species.

Overall, NTP and PAW showed effectiveness in the inactivation of MPF in food. However, the plasma operation and treatment parameters must be carefully considered to achieve the maximum efficiency offered by NTP and PAW considering MPF inactivation in food.

3.2 Direct degradation of mycotoxin

Comprehensive literature reviews on the application of NTP for the degradation of several mycotoxins in food over the past years have been discussed in previous publications, while that of PAW is still lacking [4, 28, 29, 39, 40]. This chapter highlighted the key findings from the past 3 years on the effects of NTP and PAW on the degradation of mycotoxins in food. A summary of these findings is shown in **Table 2**.

Plasma device and treatment parameters	Food matrix	Mycotoxin of concern	Key findings	Source
a. NTP treatment				
Device: DBD Gas: air Power supply: 300 W, 3500 Hz Treatment time: 0, 5, 10 min	Raw wheat grains	T-2, HT-2	• Plasma characteristics: Nitrous fumes (NO_x, NO, NO_2) = 289.50 ppm H_2O_2 = 168 ppm O_3 = 689 ppm • T-2 and HT-2 concentrations significantly decreased up to 79.80 and 70.40%, respectively, after 10 min of air-NTP treatment	Iqdiam et al. [41]
Device: LP-DBD plasma reactor Gas: O_2, N_2 5.0, Ar 5.0, synthetic air Power supply: 6 W, 25 kHz, 2.50 kV Treatment time: 10, 20, 30 min	Oat flour	T-2, HT-2	• Maximum T-2 reduction was 44.42% after 30 min of treatment using N_2 gas • Maximum HT-2 reduction was 40.87% after 30 min of treatment using N_2 gas	Kiš et al. [42]
Device: SBD Gas: ambient air Gas flow rate: 1 L/min Power supply: 0.18 (low) and 0.31 (high) W/cm discharge power Treatment time: 0.50, 1, 2, 4, 8 min	Corn kernels	AFB1	• 100% decontamination of AFB1 was achieved after 4 min of treatment with high discharge power operation of SBD plasma	Hojnik et al. [43]
Device: DBD-ACP Gas: humid air Power supply: 300 W Distance from electrode to sample: 2 mm Treatment time: 0, 2, 4, 6, 8, 10 min	Raw barley grains	DON	• Plasma characteristics: O_3 = 675 ppm H_2O_2 = 200 ppm NO_x = 480 ppm • Maximum DON degradation of 54.4% was achieved after 10 min of ACP treatment • Changing the moisture content of barley did not produce significant differences in DON degradation levels • DON degradation significantly increased when barley grains were steeped without subsequent drying prior to ACP treatment	Feizollahi et al. [44]

Plasma device and treatment parameters	Food matrix	Mycotoxin of concern	Key findings	Source
Device: AP plasma jet generated from a pulsed DBD jet Gas: He Gas flow rate: 2 standard L/min Distance from plasma jet outlet to sample: 12 mm Power supply: 20 kHz, 6 kV Treatment time: 10 min	Maize	AFB1, FB1	• AFB1 and FB1 on maize samples were reduced by 65 and 64%, respectively, after 10 min of plasma exposure • Degradation byproducts were only detected in AFB1 for maize samples, with AFB1-dihydrodiol as the most prominent degraded product	Wielogorska et al. [45]
Device: plasma jet Gas: compressed air Gas flow rate: 107 L/min Power supply: 650 W, 70–90 kHz, 4.40 kV Distance from the nozzle to sample: 5 cm Treatment time: 0.50, 1, 1.50, 2 min (constant treatment), and 3, 4, 5 min (agitated treatment)	Unroasted raw peanuts	AFB1, AFB2	• 2 min of constant APPJ treatment reduced total aflatoxin (AFB1 + AFB2) by 23%, while 5 min of agitated APPJ treatment reduced total aflatoxin by 38%	Iqdiam et al. [46]
Device: RDBD Gas: commercial He Gas flow rate: 1.50 L/min Power supply: 30 W, 850 V Treatment time: 0, 1, 4, 8, 10, 12, 16, 20, 24, 30 min	Roasted ground coffee	OTA	• 30 min of NTP exposure reduced OTA by approximately 50%	Casas-Junco et al. [35]

Plasma device and treatment parameters	Food matrix	Mycotoxin of concern	Key findings	Source
b. PAW treatment				
Device: nonthermal AP plasma jet Gas: air Gas flow rate: 8 L/min Power supply: 4.40 kV Water source: distilled water (100 mL) PAW activation time: 20 min Duration: 0, 5, 10, 15, 20 min	Raw and germinating barley	DON	• PAW characteristics: pH = 2.80 EC[a] = 451.50 μS/cm ORP[b] = 463.80 mV • 20 min of PAW treatment resulted in a maximum reduction of DON by 25.80 and 38.30% in raw and germinating barley, respectively	Chen et al. [47]

[a] *Electrical conductivity.*
[b] *Oxidation-reduction potential.*

Table 2.
Recent findings on the effects of gaseous NTP and PAW treatments on mycotoxin degradation in food.

Among the mycotoxins, the aflatoxins are regarded as one of the most widely distributed and toxic mycotoxins, and the International Agency for Research on Cancer has categorized AFB1, AFB2, AFG1, and AFG2 as Group 1 carcinogens [48, 49]. Thus, most of the research on mycotoxin degradation using NTP has focused on aflatoxins, especially on AFB1. A recent study has shown that AFB1 was completely degraded in corn kernels after treatment for only 4 min with a high discharge power operation of a surface barrier discharge (SBD) system in ambient air [43]. By contrast, a similar study reported a low reduction (65%) of AFB1 in maize after treatment with an AP plasma jet using He as the feed gas for 10 min [45]. The same author also reported a comparable reduction of 64% of fumonisin B1 (FB1) using the same treatment conditions [45]. Meanwhile, short treatment periods of 2–5 min corresponding to constant (peanuts placed directly under the plasma jet flame) and agitated (peanuts placed in a moving conveyor belt) air plasma jet surface treatments reduced the total aflatoxin levels (AFB1 + AFB2) by only 23 and 38%, respectively [46]. T-2 and HT-2, which are trichothecene mycotoxins of the *Fusarium* species, are also commonly studied in recent years. Iqdiam et al. [41] reported that T-2 and HT-2 concentrations in wheat grains significantly decreased up to 79.80 and 70.40%, respectively, after 10 min of air-NTP treatment using a DBD system. Kiš et al. [42] also used an LP-DBD plasma reactor for T-2 and HT-2 degradation in oat flour and achieved relatively low maximum reductions of T-2 (44.42%) and HT-2 (40.87%) after 30 min of treatment using N_2 gas. Additionally, DON in raw barley grains was degraded by 54.40% after 10 min of DBD atmospheric cold plasma (ACP) treatment with air as feed gas [44], which is lower compared with T-2 and HT-2 reductions using similar treatment conditions [41]. Meanwhile, the degradation of 50% of ochratoxin A (OTA) in roasted ground coffee took 30 min of NTP exposure with an RDBD using He gas [35]. Overall, NTP treatment demonstrated the effectiveness of up to 100% of mycotoxin degradation in food but with a large variation. Furthermore, the results from these studies imply that the type of plasma device, feed gas, treatment duration, type of mycotoxin, and food matrix may affect the efficiency of NTP treatment for mycotoxin degradation in food.

Meanwhile, the effect of PAW on the degradation of mycotoxins in food is less studied compared with NTP treatment. In recent years, only one research has shown the applicability of PAW for mycotoxin degradation in the food matrix. Chen et al. [47] demonstrated that 20 min of treatment with PAW generated using a nonthermal AP plasma jet from the air and distilled water resulted in maximum reductions of DON by 25.80 and 38.30% in raw and germinating barley, respectively. This phenomenon may have resulted in less interest in PAW compared to NTP due to the low mycotoxin degradation capability of PAW. Therefore, further research on the use of PAW for mycotoxin degradation is necessary to be optimized for decontamination of food from harmful mycotoxins.

4. Mechanisms of action of NTP and PAW in mycotoxin decontamination of food

4.1 Proposed mechanism of MPF inactivation

The mechanisms involved in the plasma-induced inactivation of MPF have been thoroughly discussed in past literature [30, 50]. The reactive species produced during NTP and PAW generation are generally believed to contribute substantially to the action of these technologies against different microorganisms, including bacteria and fungi [38, 50, 51]. Particularly, the action of ROS in MPF inactivation has been elucidated in many studies, while that of RNS remains unknown [52].

The harsh oxidative environment of NTP and/or PAW can result in fungal spore inactivation through denaturation of the proteins that comprise the coating of spores, thus leading to the loss of spore coat integrity, which then exposes the center of the spore to plasma ROS [28, 31]. The destruction of spore coat integrity results in the reduction of cell viability [31]. For instance, the disintegration of the cell walls of *A. flavus* and *A. parasiticus* spores led to the release of cytoplasmic structures as clusters following atmospheric NTP treatment [36]. Similarly, the walls of *A. brassicicola* spores had morphological changes, such as breakage or leakage of the outer membranes, following PAW treatment [38]. The authors concluded that the spores of *A. brassicicola* lost their integrity, and the contents of the cells dispersed into clusters as observed in scanning electron microscopy images [38]. In addition, the acidic environment of PAW could affect the cell walls of spores [36]. For instance, a recent study concluded that the inactivation of *A. flavus* spore was due to the synergistic effects of acidified PAW environment and long-lived reactive species [53]. In addition to the denaturation of the spore coat proteins, MPF inactivation may also occur by damaging the lipid bilayers, which results in a ruptured fungal cell wall [28, 31]. The core of the spore becomes vulnerable again to attacks by the plasma reactive species once the cell wall is ruptured, leading to fungal inactivation [28, 31]. Other mechanisms involved in the damage of fungal spores are the accumulation of charged particles and continuous bombardment of reactive species on the external surface of spores, which both lead to cell wall rupture [31]. Reports indicate that the accumulated charged particles resulted in the formation of enlarged pores on the spore surface of *A. flavus* and *A. parasiticus* after NTP treatment due to electroporation, which promotes spore death [54].

Thus far, the mechanisms of MPF inactivation using plasma treatments involve changes in fungi morphology. However, the morphology of *F. oxysporum* spore was not altered after its inactivation using NTP treatment [50]. The authors reported that the increase in lipid accumulation inside the cells induced apoptosis, which is a form of programmed cell death [50]. Considering the direct action of select ROS on MPF inactivation, previous literature suggested that the action of •OH radicals on unsaturated fatty acids and the oxidation of amino acids can respectively lead to lipid peroxidation and protein oxidation, which can result in fungi death [30]. Furthermore, the interaction of oxygen radicals with DNA can lead to the formation of base adducts, resulting in DNA oxidation, which can also cause fungi death [30].

Summarizing the results of the above-mentioned studies, the MPF inactivation of plasma mainly occurs due to changes in the morphology caused by the damage in the protective coating of the fungal spores, membrane peroxidation and leakage, protein oxidation, DNA damage, and apoptosis [4, 30]. Notably, the observed and proposed mechanisms of MPF inactivation by the aforementioned studies may have varied due to the different plasma devices and processing parameters employed in the individual studies, which can lead to different actions of NTP and/or PAW against MPF inactivation.

4.2 Proposed mechanism of mycotoxin degradation

The mechanisms of mycotoxin degradation induced by NTP treatments have been comprehensively reported elsewhere [28, 40, 51]. AFB1 is the major mycotoxin that is studied in plasma investigations; thus, the reports on the mechanism of mycotoxin degradation induced by plasma mainly revolved around AFB1 [55]. The toxicity of AFB1, and aflatoxins in general, is related to the C8 = C9 double bond on the furan ring, which is considered to be the toxicity site [55]. Generally, the degradation of AFB1 is proposed to have resulted from the action of long-lived ROS with chemical structures of AFB1, particularly at the toxicity site [52, 56]. For example, reports indicated that O_3 and •OH radical were among the primary contributors to the degradation of AFB1 into six major degradation byproducts using DBD-based plasma treatment, and the authors provided an illustration of the proposed degradation mechanism in their work [52]. The authors proposed the following two mechanisms of degradation—(1) an addition reaction involving H_2O, H, or CHO radicals and (2) an epoxidation reaction involving HO_2• and oxidation reactions, including O_3, H_2O_2, and •OH radical [52]. An earlier study also proposed that the O•, H•, and •OH radicals produced from a low-temperature RF plasma were the major reactive species that degraded AFB1 into five major degradation byproducts, and two mechanisms of degradation were introduced [57]. Overall, the two studies revealed that the degradation of AFB1 begins with the breakage of the C8 = C9 double bonds on the furan ring, followed by an attack by the ROS, thus resulting in the formation of AFB1 degradation byproducts [52, 57]. This conclusion was further confirmed in a recent study, which investigated the degradation byproducts of AFB1 using an atmospheric pressure plasma jet generated from a pulsed DBD jet, stating that AFB1 degradation byproducts are produced from the modifications at the furan ring [45].

The degradation of other major mycotoxins, such as OTA, could also be mainly due to ROS molecules and radicals, such as O_3, H_2O_2, and •OH radical, as well as UV irradiation and etching [35]. The ROS could promote the degradation of OTA into slightly toxic compounds, such as L-phenylalanine [35]. Furthermore, the degradation byproducts of ZEN following a plasma jet-based NTP treatment were reported, which identified two degradation byproducts [45].

Studies on the mechanism of action for mycotoxin degradation using PAW treatment and determination of mycotoxin degradation byproducts post-treatment are currently unavailable. However, similar to the gaseous NTP, the different ROS dominates the degradation of mycotoxins during PAW treatment. For example, the H_2O_2, O_3, and nitrate ion (NO_3^-) reactive species were believed to be the major reason for DON degradation in barley during PAW treatment [47].

Overall, the reactive species are the major contributors to the degradation of mycotoxins during NTP treatment of food. Further work on the elucidation of degradation mechanism and byproducts of other major mycotoxins, such as OTA, DON, or ZEN, following NTP treatment, is also needed. Moreover, extensive research on the degradation byproducts of these mycotoxins and proposed mechanisms using PAW treatment is warranted.

5. Effects of NTP and PAW treatments on food quality

In addition to the effective and significant decontamination of food from mycotoxins using NTP and PAW treatments, another known promising characteristic of these technologies is the retainment or negligible impact on the nutritional and other key properties of food. This chapter emphasizes the effects of NTP and PAW treatments on food quality following mycotoxin decontamination from the most recent studies.

Results revealed that the overall likeability was positively correlated with the overall texture (r = 0.77) and flavor (r = 0.87) of peanuts [46]. Generally, NTP treatment did not produce a negative effect on the sensory properties of food [34, 46]. For example, the treatment of red pepper flakes for *A. flavus* inactivation did not significantly affect its color and flavor properties compared with the control [34]. Similarly, the overall appearance of peanuts after NTP treatment using a plasma jet device did not significantly change, while the overall likeability, flavor, and texture of the NTP-treated peanuts significantly increased; this finding indicates that NTP treatment can also enhance the sensory characteristics of peanuts [46].

By contrast, plasma treatments had varying effects on the physicochemical properties of food. NTP treatment of pistachio nuts for *A. flavus* inactivation revealed a slight increase in the antioxidant activity and a significant increase in malondialdehyde values, while the total phenolic content remained unchanged; however, a decrease in chlorophyll, total carotenoid, and color parameters was observed [31]. NTP treatment was also found to significantly lower the capsaicin and ascorbic acid levels of red pepper flakes, but its antioxidant activity and color were unaffected by the treatment [34]. Similarly, the color of wheat grains did not also show changes after NTP treatment, along with the nitrogen, protein, starch, and moisture contents [41]. Another study also reported the absence of significant differences in the moisture, protein, and β-glucan contents of barley after NTP treatment compared with control [44]. The peanut oil extracted from NTP-treated peanuts also had no significant difference in its peroxide value, free fatty acid, acidity value, and oxidative stability index compared with control after the treatment [46]. Meanwhile, the NTP treatment of corn kernels and peanuts produced slight oxidation and bitterness in taste [43, 46]. By contrast, PAW treatment did not affect the overall quality of Chinese kale seeds [38].

Overall, the effects of NTP and PAW treatments on food quality may differ depending on the processing parameters employed and the type of food matrix tested [11].

6. Safety of mycotoxin degradation byproducts in treated food after NTP and PAW treatments

Examining the safety or toxicity of the food post-treatment and the byproducts produced during the process is important for any emerging technology, especially in the field of food processing. However, investigations regarding these concerns in the field of plasma research for mycotoxin decontamination are still limited in the current state of literature. The AFB1 byproducts are hypothesized to have reduced toxicity due to the loss of the C8 = C9 double bond, which is related to its toxicity [57]. This finding was confirmed in a recent study, which reported that the degradation byproducts of AFB1 after AP plasma jet treatment showed no increased cytotoxicity in human hepatocarcinoma (HepG2) cells [45]. Additionally, another study revealed through a brine shrimp (*Artemia salina*) lethality bioassay that the OTA extract from untreated coffee was "toxic," which corresponds to a 50–88.30% mortality in brine shrimp larvae [35]. However, the mortality rate was reduced to "slightly toxic" levels (10–33.33% mortality) when OTA extract from NTP-treated coffee was exposed to brine shrimp larvae [35]. Meanwhile, the safety or toxicity of the original food that has undergone NTP or PAW treatment for mycotoxin decontamination has not been currently assessed.

Overall, the current investigations demonstrate that NTP treatment can degrade mycotoxins and produce degradation byproducts that are nontoxic or with lower degrees of toxicity compared with the toxic parent compound. However, the safety of the food treated with NTP or PAW remains unknown. Hence, future research should address this issue to guarantee the safety of plasma-treated food for human consumption.

7. Conclusions

The nonthermal-based treatments such as NTP and PAW have shown promising results in the field of food decontamination against biological and chemical contaminants. Particularly, their effects on decontaminating foods from mycotoxins have been exceptional, and the capability of NTP and PAW to inactivate fungi and degrade mycotoxins is due to the oxidizing capacities of the existing reactive species in the plasma. The existing literature reveals that NTP and PAW inactivated the fungi that produce the mycotoxins as well as degraded the mycotoxins in foods, such as nuts, seeds, and spices, without producing harmful byproducts and having mild impacts on food quality. However, the result is still inconsistent in all studies. For instance, the current literature indicates NTP as the better treatment option for MPF inactivation and mycotoxin degradation compared with PAW. This finding is due to the desirable inactivation or degradation efficiencies of NTP treatment of up to 100% in no longer than 30 min, whereas low efficiencies of PAW treatment were observed and can only be achieved at long treatments. However, NTP treatment is more prone to induce undesirable effects on food quality compared with PAW.

Overall, the decontamination of foods from mycotoxins using NTP and PAW treatments and their effects on food quality is dependent on many factors, including the plasma device, the treatment parameters (such as power supply, type of feed gas, and treatment duration), the fungi species, the type of mycotoxin, and the food matrix. Thus, comparison of the results from various studies is difficult due to this diversity in plasma operation techniques. Therefore, deciding which NTP or PAW treatment is the best for mycotoxin decontamination of food remains unclear. Hence, consideration and optimization of the results from the current studies are crucial to ensure maximum utilization of NTP and PAW technologies for mycotoxin decontamination of food.

Author details

Hsiu-Ling Chen[1*], Rachelle D. Arcega[1], Samuel Herianto[2,3,4], Chih-Yao Hou[5] and Chia-Min Lin[5]

1 Department of Food Safety/Hygiene and Risk Management, College of Medicine, National Cheng Kung University, Tainan, Taiwan

2 Chemical Biology and Molecular Biophysics Program, Taiwan International Graduate Program (TIGP), Academia Sinica, Taipei, Taiwan

3 Institute of Chemistry, Academia Sinica, Taipei, Taiwan

4 Department of Chemistry (Chemical Biology Division), College of Science, National Taiwan University, Taipei, Taiwan

5 Department of Seafood Science, College of Hydrosphere, National Kaohsiung University of Science and Technology, Kaohsiung, Taiwan

*Address all correspondence to: hsiulinchen@mail.ncku.edu.tw

References

[1] Liew WPP, Mohd-Redzwan S. Mycotoxin: Its impact on gut health and microbiota. Frontiers in Cellular and Infection Microbiology. 2018;**8**:60. DOI: 10.3389/fcimb.2018.00060

[2] Awuchi CG, Ondari EN, Ogbonna CU, Upadhyay AK, Baran K, Okpalam COR, et al. Mycotoxins affecting animals, foods, humans, and plants: Types, occurrence, toxicities, action mechanisms, prevention, and detoxification strategies—A revisit. Food. 2021;**10**(6):1279. DOI: 10.3390/foods10061279

[3] Enyiukwu D, Awurum A, Nwaneri J. Mycotoxins in stored agricultural products: Implications to food safety and health and prospects of plant-derived pesticides as novel approach to their management. Greener Journal of Microbiology and Antimicrobials. 2014;**2**(3):32-48. DOI: 10.15580/GJMA.2014.3.0521014241

[4] Gavahian M, Cullen P. Cold plasma as an emerging technique for mycotoxin-free food: Efficacy, mechanisms, and trends. Food Reviews International. 2020;**36**(2):193-214. DOI: 10.1080/87559129.2019.1630638

[5] Oğuz H. Mycotoxins and their importance. Turkiye Klinikleri Veterinary Sciences- Pharmacology and Toxicology. 2017;**3**(2):113-119

[6] Vila-Donat P, Marín S, Sanchis V, Ramos A. A review of the mycotoxin adsorbing agents, with an emphasis on their multi-binding capacity, for animal feed decontamination. Food and Chemical Toxicology. 2018;**114**:246-259. DOI: 10.1016/j.fct.2018.02.044

[7] Hassan FF, Hussein HZ, Hawar SN. Detection and detoxification of aflatoxin B1 from fish feedstuff using microwave and ozone gas. Ibn Al-Haitham Journal for Pure and Applied Science. 2018;**31**(1):28-36. DOI: 10.30526/31.1.1847

[8] Freitas-Silva O, Venâncio A. Ozone applications to prevent and degrade mycotoxins: A review. Drug Metabolism Reviews. 2010;**42**(4):612-620. DOI: 10.3109/03602532.2010.484461

[9] Kalagatur NK, Mudili V, Kamasani JR, Siddaiah C. Discrete and combined effects of Ylang-Ylang (*Cananga odorata*) essential oil and gamma irradiation on growth and mycotoxins production by *Fusarium graminearum* in maize. Food Control. 2018;**94**:276-283. DOI: 10.1016/j.foodcont.2018.07.030

[10] Wang B, Mahoney NE, Khir R, Wu B, Zhou C, Pan Z, et al. Degradation kinetics of aflatoxin B1 and B2 in solid medium by using pulsed light irradiation. Journal of the Science of Food and Agriculture. 2018;**98**(14):5220-5224. DOI: 10.1002/jsfa.9058

[11] Herianto S, Hou CY, Lin CM, Chen HL. Nonthermal plasma-activated water: A comprehensive review of this new tool for enhanced food safety and quality. Comprehensive Reviews in Food Science and Food Safety. 2021;**20**(1):583-626. DOI: 10.1111/1541-4337.12667

[12] Lin CM, Chu YC, Hsiao CP, Wu JS, Hsieh CW, Hou CY. The optimization of plasma-activated water treatments to inactivate *Salmonella enteritidis* (ATCC 13076) on shell eggs. Food. 2019;**8**(10):520. DOI: 10.3390/foods8100520

[13] Perinban S, Orsat V, Raghavan V. Nonthermal plasma-liquid interactions

in food processing: A review. Comprehensive Reviews in Food Science and Food Safety. 2019;**18**(6):1985-2008. DOI: 10.1111/1541-4337.12503

[14] Thirumdas R, Kothakota A, Annapure U, Siliveru K, Blundell R, Gatt R, et al. Plasma activated water (PAW): Chemistry, physico-chemical properties, applications in food and agriculture. Trends in Food Science & Technology. 2018;**77**:21-31. DOI: 10.1016/j.tifs.2018.05.007

[15] Zhou R, Zhou R, Wang P, Xian Y, Mai-Prochnow A, Lu X, et al. Plasma-activated water: Generation, origin of reactive species and biological applications. Journal of Physics D: Applied Physics. 2020;**53**(30):303001. DOI: 10.1088/1361-6463/ab81cf

[16] Holubová Ľ, Kyzek S, Ďurovcová I, Fabová J, Horváthová E, Ševčovičová A, et al. Non-thermal plasma—A new green priming agent for plants? International Journal of Molecular Sciences. 2020; **21**(24):9466. DOI: 10.3390/ijms21249466

[17] Zhou R, Zhou R, Prasad K, Fang Z, Speight R, Bazaka K, et al. Cold atmospheric plasma activated water as a prospective disinfectant: The crucial role of peroxynitrite. Green Chemistry. 2018;**20**(23):5276-5284. DOI: 10.1039/C8GC02800A

[18] Bourke P, Ziuzina D, Han L, Cullen P, Gilmore BF. Microbiological interactions with cold plasma. Journal of Applied Microbiology. 2017;**123**(2):308-324. DOI: 10.1111/jam.13429

[19] Nascimento FD, Moshkalev S, Machida M. Changes in properties of dielectric barrier discharge plasma jets for different gases and for insulating and conducting transfer plates. Brazilian Journal of Physics. 2017;**47**:278-287. DOI: 10.1007/s13538-017-0492-1

[20] Zheng Y, Wu S, Dang J, Wang S, Liu Z, Fang J, et al. Reduction of phoxim pesticide residues from grapes by atmospheric pressure non-thermal air plasma activated water. Journal of Hazardous Materials. 2019;**377**:98-105. DOI: 10.1016/j.jhazmat.2019.05.058

[21] Simpson BK, Nollet LM, Toldrá F, Benjakul S, Paliyath G, Hui Y. Food Biochemistry and Food Processing. Hoboken, NJ: John Wiley & Sons; 2012

[22] Martínez MC, Andriantsitohaina R. Reactive nitrogen species: Molecular mechanisms and potential significance in health and disease. Antioxidants & Redox Signaling. 2009;**11**(3):669-702. DOI: 10.1089/ars.2007.1993

[23] López M, Calvo T, Prieto M, Múgica-Vidal R, Muro-Fraguas I, Alba-Elías F, et al. A review on non-thermal atmospheric plasma for food preservation: Mode of action, determinants of effectiveness, and applications. Frontiers in Microbiology. 2019;**10**:622. DOI: 10.3389/fmicb.2019.00622

[24] Lin CM, Herianto S, Chen HL, Chiu YC, Hou CY. The application of a novel non-thermal plasma device with double rotary plasma jets for inactivation of *Salmonella* Enteritidis on shell eggs and its effects on sensory properties. International Journal of Food Microbiology. 2021;**355**:109332. DOI: 10.1016/j.ijfoodmicro.2021.109332

[25] Lin CM, Herianto S, Syu SM, Song CH, Chen HL, Hou CY. Applying a large-scale device using non-thermal plasma for microbial decontamination on shell eggs and its effects on the sensory characteristics. LWT. 2021;**142**:111067. DOI: 10.1016/j.lwt.2021.111067

[26] Hou CY, Lai YC, Hsiao CP, Chen SY, Liu CT, Wu JS, et al. Antibacterial

activity and the physicochemical characteristics of plasma activated water on tomato surfaces. LWT. 2021;**149**:111879. DOI: 10.1016/j.lwt.2021.111879

[27] Lin CM, Hsiao CP, Lin HS, Liou JS, Hsieh CW, Wu JS, et al. The antibacterial efficacy and mechanism of plasma-activated water against *Salmonella* Enteritidis (ATCC 13076) on shell eggs. Food. 2020;**9**(10):1491. DOI: 10.3390/foods9101491

[28] Misra N, Yadav B, Roopesh M, Jo C. Cold plasma for effective fungal and mycotoxin control in foods: Mechanisms, inactivation effects, and applications. Comprehensive Reviews in Food Science and Food Safety. 2019;**18**(1):106-120. DOI: 10.1111/1541-4337.12398

[29] Gavahian M, Sheu SC, Magnani M, Mousavi KA. Emerging technologies for mycotoxins removal from foods: Recent advances, roles in sustainable food consumption, and strategies for industrial applications. Journal of Food Processing and Preservation. 2021;**00**:e15922. DOI: 10.1111/jfpp.15922

[30] Mravlje J, Regvar M, Vogel-Mikuš K. Development of cold plasma technologies for surface decontamination of seed fungal pathogens: Present status and perspectives. Journal of Fungi. 2021;**7**(8):650. DOI: 10.3390/jof7080650

[31] Makari M, Hojjati M, Shahbazi S, Askari H. Elimination of *Aspergillus flavus* from pistachio nuts with dielectric barrier discharge (DBD) cold plasma and its impacts on biochemical indices. Journal of Food Quality. 2021:9968711. DOI: 10.1155/2021/9968711

[32] Lee Y, Lee YY, Kim YS, Balaraju K, Mok YS, Yoo SJ, et al. Enhancement of seed germination and microbial disinfection on ginseng by cold plasma treatment. Journal of Ginseng Research. 2021;**45**(4):519-526. DOI: 10.1016/j.jgr.2020.12.002

[33] Ghorashi A, Tasouji MR, Kargarian A. Optimum cold plasma generating device for treatment of *Aspergillus flavus* from nuts surface. Journal of Food Science and Technology. 2020;**57**:3988-3994. DOI: 10.1007/s13197-020-04429-y

[34] Kim JE, Oh YJ, Song AY, Min SC. Preservation of red pepper flakes using microwave-combined cold plasma treatment. Journal of the Science of Food and Agriculture. 2019;**99**(4):1577-1585. DOI: 10.1002/jsfa.9336

[35] Casas-Junco PP, Solís-Pacheco JR, Ragazzo-Sánchez JA, Aguilar-Uscanga BR, Bautista-Rosales PU, Calderón-Santoyo M. Cold plasma treatment as an alternative for ochratoxin A detoxification and inhibition of mycotoxigenic fungi in roasted coffee. Toxins. 2019;**11**(6):337. DOI: 10.3390/toxins11060337

[36] Sen Y, Onal-Ulusoy B, Mutlu M. *Aspergillus* decontamination in hazelnuts: Evaluation of atmospheric and low-pressure plasma technology. Innovative Food Science & Emerging Technologies. 2019;**54**:235-242. DOI: 10.1016/j.ifset.2019.04.014

[37] Terebun P, Kwiatkowski M, Hensel K, Kopacki M, Pawłat J. Influence of plasma activated water generated in a gliding arc discharge reactor on germination of beetroot and carrot seeds. Applied Sciences. 2021;**11**(13):6164. DOI: 10.3390/app11136164

[38] Suwannarat S, Thammaniphit C, Srisonphan S. Electrohydraulic streamer discharge plasma-enhanced *Alternaria brassicicola* disinfection in seed sterilization. ACS Applied Materials &

Interfaces. 2021;**13**:43975-43983. DOI: 10.1021/acsami.1c10771

[39] Adebo OA, Molelekoa T, Makhuvele R, Adebiyi JA, Oyedeji AB, Gbashi S, et al. A review on novel non-thermal food processing techniques for mycotoxin reduction. International Journal of Food Science & Technology. 2021;**56**(1):13-27. DOI: 10.1111/ijfs.14734

[40] Hojnik N, Cvelbar U, Tavčar-Kalcher G, Walsh JL, Križaj I. Mycotoxin decontamination of food: Cold atmospheric pressure plasma versus "classic" decontamination. Toxins. 2017;**9**(5):151. DOI: 10.3390/toxins9050151

[41] Iqdiam BM, Feizollahi E, Arif MF, Jeganathan B, Vasanthan T, Thilakarathna MS, et al. Reduction of T-2 and HT-2 mycotoxins by atmospheric cold plasma and its impact on quality changes and germination of wheat grains. Journal of Food Science. 2021;**86**(4):1354-1371. DOI: 10.1111/1750-3841.15658

[42] Kiš M, Milošević S, Vulić A, Herceg Z, Vukušić T, Pleadin J. Efficacy of low pressure DBD plasma in the reduction of T-2 and HT-2 toxin in oat flour. Food Chemistry. 2020;**316**:126372. DOI: 10.1016/j.foodchem.2020.126372

[43] Hojnik N, Modic M, Žigon D, Kovač J, Jurov A, Dickenson A, et al. Cold atmospheric pressure plasma-assisted removal of aflatoxin B1 from contaminated corn kernels. Plasma Processes and Polymers. 2021;**18**(1):2000163. DOI: 10.1002/ppap.202000163

[44] Feizollahi E, Iqdiam B, Vasanthan T, Thilakarathna MS, Roopesh M. Effects of atmospheric-pressure cold plasma treatment on deoxynivalenol degradation, quality parameters, and germination of barley grains. Applied Sciences. 2020;**10**(10):3530. DOI: 10.3390/app10103530

[45] Wielogorska E, Ahmed Y, Meneely J, Graham WG, Elliott CT, Gilmore BF. A holistic study to understand the detoxification of mycotoxins in maize and impact on its molecular integrity using cold atmospheric plasma treatment. Food Chemistry. 2019;**301**:125281. DOI: 10.1016/j.foodchem.2019.125281

[46] Iqdiam BM, Abuagela MO, Boz Z, Marshall SM, Goodrich-Schneider R, Sims CA, et al. Effects of atmospheric pressure plasma jet treatment on aflatoxin level, physiochemical quality, and sensory attributes of peanuts. Journal of Food Processing and Preservation. 2020;**44**(1):e14305. DOI: 10.1111/jfpp.14305

[47] Chen D, Chen P, Cheng Y, Peng P, Liu J, Ma Y, et al. Deoxynivalenol decontamination in raw and germinating barley treated by plasma-activated water and intense pulsed light. Food and Bioprocess Technology. 2019;**12**(2):246-254. DOI: 10.1007/s11947-018-2206-2

[48] Pitt JI, Miller JD. A concise history of mycotoxin research. Journal of Agricultural and Food Chemistry. 2017;**65**(33):7021-7033. DOI: 10.1021/acs.jafc.6b04494

[49] Bhat R, Rai RV, Karim AA. Mycotoxins in food and feed: Present status and future concerns. Comprehensive Reviews in Food Science and Food Safety. 2010;**9**(1):57-81. DOI: 10.1111/j.1541-4337.2009.00094.x

[50] Panngom K, Lee SH, Park DH, Sim GB, Kim YH, Uhm HS, et al. Non-thermal plasma treatment diminishes fungal viability and up-regulates resistance genes in a plant host. PLoS

One. 2014;**9**(6):e99300. DOI: 10.1371/journal.pone.0099300

[51] Mravlje J, Regvar M, Starič P, Mozetič M, Vogel-Mikuš K. Cold plasma affects germination and fungal community structure of buckwheat seeds. Plants. 2021;**10**(5):851. DOI: 10.3390/plants10050851

[52] Shi H, Cooper B, Stroshine RL, Ileleji KE, Keener KM. Structures of degradation products and degradation pathways of aflatoxin B1 by high-voltage atmospheric cold plasma (HVACP) treatment. Journal of Agricultural and Food Chemistry. 2017;**65**(30):6222-6230. DOI: 10.1021/acs.jafc.7b01604

[53] Los A, Ziuzina D, Boehm D, Cullen PJ, Bourke P. Inactivation efficacies and mechanisms of gas plasma and plasma-activated water against *Aspergillus flavus* spores and biofilms: A comparative study. Applied and Environmental Microbiology. 2020;**86**(9):e02619-e02619. DOI: 10.1128/AEM.02619-19

[54] Devi Y, Thirumdas R, Sarangapani C, Deshmukh R, Annapure U. Influence of cold plasma on fungal growth and aflatoxins production on groundnuts. Food Control. 2017;**77**:187-191. DOI: 10.1016/j.foodcont.2017.02.019

[55] Wu Y, Cheng JH, Sun DW. Blocking and degradation of aflatoxins by cold plasma treatments: Applications and mechanisms. Trends in Food Science & Technology. 2021;**109**:647-661. DOI: 10.1016/j.tifs.2021.01.053

[56] Sakudo A, Toyokawa Y, Misawa T, Imanishi Y. Degradation and detoxification of aflatoxin B1 using nitrogen gas plasma generated by a static induction thyristor as a pulsed power supply. Food Control. 2017;**73**:619-626. DOI: 10.1016/j.foodcont.2016.09.014

[57] Wang SQ, Huang GQ, Li YP, Xiao JX, Zhang Y, Jiang WL. Degradation of aflatoxin B 1 by low-temperature radio frequency plasma and degradation product elucidation. European Food Research and Technology. 2015;**241**(1):103-113. DOI: 10.1007/s00217-015-2439-5